The Simple 5 Ingre
Keto Cookbook
Delicious & Easy Ketogenic Diet Recipes for Healthy & Fast Meals

By Sydney Foster

© 2018

© Copyright 2018 by CiJiRO Publishing- All rights reserved.

This document is geared toward providing exact and reliable information in regard to the topic and issue covered. The publication is sold with the idea that the publisher is not required to render accounting, officially permitted, or otherwise, qualified services. If advice is necessary, legal or professional, a practiced individual in the profession should be ordered.

- From a Declaration of Principles which was accepted and approved equally by a Committee of the American Bar Association and a Committee of Publishers and Associations.

In no way is it legal to reproduce, duplicate, or transmit any part of this document in either electronic means or in printed format. Recording of this publication is strictly prohibited and any storage of this document is not allowed unless with written permission from the publisher. All rights reserved.

The information provided herein is stated to be truthful and consistent, in that any liability, in terms of inattention or otherwise, by any usage or abuse of any policies, processes, or directions contained within is the solitary and utter responsibility of the recipient reader. Under no circumstances will any legal responsibility or blame be held against the publisher for any reparation, damages, or monetary loss due to the information herein, either directly or indirectly.

Respective authors own all copyrights not held by the publisher.

The information herein is offered for informational purposes solely, and is universal as so. The presentation of the information is without contract or any type of guarantee assurance.

The trademarks that are used are without any consent, and the publication of the trademark is without permission or backing by the trademark owner. All trademarks and brands within this book are for clarifying purposes only and are the owned by the owners themselves, not affiliated with this document.

Sign Up for Free Weekly Recipes, Tips and Tricks and more at:

http://www.KetoDiet.coach

Table of Contents

Introduction 11

Chapter 1: Breakfast Recipes 13

Keto Coffee 13

Peanut Butter & Chocolate Smoothies 14

Chia & Blackberry Pudding 15

Sage & Strawberry Smoothie 16

Breakfast Roll Ups 17

Angel Eggs 18

Chocolate & Strawberry Smoothie 19

Frozen Coffee 20

Keto Porridge 21

Macadamia & Salted Chocolate Smoothie 22

Bacon & Cheddar Omelet 23

Bacon & Eggs 24

Eggs Benedict 25

Spanakopita 26

Green Berry Smoothie 27

Cinnamon Smoothie 28

Breakfast Bake 29

Peanut Butter Cup Smoothie 30

Pesto Scrambled Eggs 31

Chapter 2: Lunch Recipes 33

Basil & Tomato Soup 33

Caprese Salad 34

Garlic Monkey Bread 35

Cheesy Mug Melt 36

BLT Salad 37

Mug Lasagna 38

Roasted Brussel Sprout Salad 39

Green Spring Salad ... 40
Taco Soup ... 41
Bacon Hot Dogs ... 42
Egg Drop Soup ... 43
Goat Cheese Salad ... 44
Avocado Salad ... 45
Broccoli & Cheese Soup ... 46

Chapter 3: Snack Recipes ... 47
Smoked Salmon Fat Bombs ... 47
Bacon Smokies ... 48
Pepper & Bacon Fat Bombs ... 49
Parmesan Chips ... 50
Burger Bacon Bombs ... 51
Pesto Mushrooms ... 52
Pizza Fat Bombs ... 53
Pimento Cheese Dip ... 54
Pork Bites ... 55
Kale Chips ... 56
Spicy Tuna Deviled Eggs ... 57
Jalapeno Popper Deviled Eggs ... 58
Keto Pizza Bite ... 59
Bacon Mozzarella Sticks ... 60
Chicken Liver Bites ... 61
Egg & Avocado Fat Bombs ... 62
Chocolate Dipped Bacon ... 63
Macadamia & Brazil Butter ... 64
Bacon & Egg Fat Bombs ... 65
Salmon Mousse Rolls ... 66
Layered Fried Queso ... 67
Cashew & Almond Butter ... 68
Coconut Chips ... 69
Jalapeno Poppers ... 70

Caprese Skewers 71
Butternut Squash Chips 72
Salami Pinwheels 73
Ramen Dip 74
Bacon Jalapenos 75
Dill Deviled Eggs 76
Mozzarella Pizza 77
Stuffed Portobello Mushrooms 78
Orange Celeriac Chips 79
Sour Cream Pork Rinds 80
Eggplant Chips 81
Coconut & Pecan Nut Butter 82
Spicy Zucchini Chips 83
Mushrooms 84

Chapter 4: Dinner Recipes 85
Sausage Stuffed Zucchini 85
Beef Ragu 87
Parmesan Salmon with Asparagus 88
Lemon Butter Cod 89
Sole Asiago 90
Pork Belly 91
Coconut Haddock 93
Roasted Pork Loin with Mustard Sauce 94
Cajun Snow Crab 95
Barbacoa Beef Roast 96
Bacon & Scallops 97
Goat Cheese Burgers 98
Lamb Chops 100
Pepper & Sausage Ragout 101
Chicken Quesadilla 102
Chicken Skewers & Peanut Sauce 103
Bacon Cups 104

Mississippi Pot Roast 105

Miso Salmon 106

Beef Wellington 107

Chicken Roulades with Gruyere 108

Baked Chicken Wings 110

Perfect Ribeye Steak 111

Perfect Ribeye 112

Slow Roasted Pork Shoulder 113

Spicy Blackberry Chicken Wings 114

Harissa Chicken Skewers 115

Beef & Broccoli Roast 116

Kalua Pork & Cabbage 119

Perfect Roast 120

Baked Pesto Seabass 121

Herb & Butter Pork Chops 122

Cheddar & Bacon Delight 123

Bacon Cordon Blue 124

Green Beans with Sesame Pork 125

Crockpot BBQ Ribs 126

Blue Cheese Pork Chops 127

Chapter 5: Side Dishes Recipes 129

Spicy Butter Beans 129

Blue Cheese Zoodles with Bacon 130

Buttery Mushrooms 131

Asparagus & Walnuts 132

Cheesy Brussel Sprouts 133

Creamed Spinach 134

Camembert Mushrooms 135

Bacon & Broccoli Salad 136

Roasted Broccoli 137

Parmesan Green Beans 138

Keto Mash 139

- Turnip Fries 140
- Pink Sauerkraut 141
- Braised Fennel with Lemon 142
- Bacon Snap Peas 143
- Bacon Jam Green Beans 144
- Cauliflower & Cheese Casserole 145
- Zucchini Gratin 146
- Brussel Sprouts & Bacon 147
- Prosciutto Brussel Sprouts & Leeks 148
- Pork Rind & Parmesan Green Beans 149
- Roasted Radishes in a Butter Sauce 150

Chapter 6: Dessert Recipes 151
- Coffee Popsicles 151
- Easy Chocolate Mousse 152
- Berry Ice Popsicles 153
- Keto Root Beer Float 154
- Easy Strawberry Shake 155
- Chocolate & Mint Ice Cream 156
- Easy Peanut Butter Cookies 158
- Lime & Strawberry Popsicles 159
- Avocado & Chocolate Pudding 160
- Lemonade Fat Bomb 161
- Fudge Popsicles 162
- Easy Strawberry Bark 163
- Toffee Nut Cups 164
- Very Berry Cheesecake Fat Bombs 165
- Pecan & Berry Mascarpone Bowl 166
- Creamy Orange Soda Float 167
- Easy Chocolate Shake 168
- Meringue Cookies 169
- Crust Free Pumpkin Cheesecake Bites 170
- Peanut Butter Fat Bomb 171

Strawberry Cheesecake Mousse 172

Peanut Butter & Coconut Balls 173

Crust Free Cheesecake Bites 174

Cholate Mouse Tropical Bites 175

Pumpkin Fudge 176

Conclusion 177

Introduction

The ketogenic diet helps many people to lose weight in no time at all, but many people fear that it's too complicated. With these five ingredient or less recipes, the ketogenic diet is easy to start and stick to. There's no reason that your meals should be time consuming, and your ingredients should never break the bank. It's easy to start your ketogenic journey. Just pick a recipe, make a short shopping list, and get started to reach your diet and health goals!

Chapter 1: Breakfast Recipes

Keto Coffee

If you'd like to add a little more oomph into your morning coffee a lot of people like to add in a teaspoon of cinnamon!

Serves: 1

Time: 10 Minutes

Calories: 463

Protein: 1 Gram

Fat: 51 Grams

Fiber: 0 Grams

Net Carbs: 0

Ingredients:

- 2 Tablespoons Ghee
- 2 Tablespoons MCT Oil Powder
- 1 ½ Cups Coffee, Hot

Directions:

1. Start by pouring your coffee into a blender, and then add in your oil powder and butter.
2. Blend until frothy, and serve immediately.

Peanut Butter & Chocolate Smoothies

Serves: 1

Time: 5 Minutes

Calories: 604

Proteins: 33 Grams

Fiber: 2 Grams

Fat: 24 Grams

Net Carbs: 6 Grams

Ingredients:

- 1 Cup Water
- 1/3 Cup Heavy Whipping Cream
- 1/3 Cup Chocolate Whey Protein Powder, Low Carb
- 2 Ice Cubes
- 2 Tablespoons Peanut Butter

Directions:

1. Blend everything together until smooth.

Chia & Blackberry Pudding

Serves: 2

Time: 45 Minutes

Calories: 437

Protein: 8 Grams

Fat: 38 Grams

Fiber: 15 Grams

Net Carbs: 8

Ingredients:

- ¼ Cup Chia Seeds
- ½ Cup Blackberries, Fresh
- 1 Teaspoon Liquid Sweetener
- 1 Cup Coconut Milk, Full Fat & Unsweetened
- 1 Teaspoon Vanilla Extract

Directions:

1. Take your vanilla, liquid sweetener and coconut milk, processing it in a blender until it begins to thicken. Add in your blackberries, processing until smooth.
2. Divide your mixture between cups, and then refrigerate for at least a half hour or up to three days.

Sage & Strawberry Smoothie

Serves: 1

Time: 5 Minutes

Calories: 173

Protein: 2 Grams

Fiber: 1 Gram

Fat: 12 Grams

Net Carbs: 5 Grams

Ingredients:

- 1 Cup Coconut Milk, Unsweetened
- 5 Strawberries, Frozen
- 1 Sage Leaf, Fresh
- 1 Teaspoon Vanilla Bean Sweetener, Sugar Free
- 2 Tablespoons Heavy Whipping Cream

Directions:

1. Blend everything together until smooth.

Breakfast Roll Ups

Serves: 5

Time: 30 Minutes

Calories: 412

Protein: 28.21 Grams

Fiber: 0 Grams

Fat: 31.66 Grams

Net Carbs: 2.26 Grams

Ingredients:

- 5 Slices Bacon, Cooked
- 5 Patties Breakfast Sausage, Cooked
- 1 ½ Cups Cheddar Cheese, Shredded
- Sea Salt to Taste
- 10 Eggs, Large

Directions:

1. Start by heating a skillet over medium-high heat, and then whisk two of your eggs together in a bowl.
2. Once your skillet is hot, then turn the heat to medium-low before adding in your eggs. Season with sea salt, and then cover the lid. Allow them to cook until the eggs are cooked almost all the way.
3. Sprinkle 1/3 cup of your cheese over it, and then lay down a strip of bacon, breaking a sausage patty in half and then place it on top.
4. Roll your egg over the filling to old, and then repeat until you're out of eggs.
5. Serve warm.

Angel Eggs

Serves: 2

Time: 30 Minutes

Calories: 184

Protein: 12 Grams

Fat: 15 Grams

Fiber: 0 Grams

Net Carbs: 1

Ingredients:

- 4 Eggs, Hardboiled & Peeled
- 1 Tablespoon Vanilla Bean Sweetener, Sugar Free
- 2 Tablespoons Mayonnaise
- 1/8 Teaspoon Cinnamon

Directions:

1. Start by halving your eggs, and then scoop out the yolk. Place it in a bowl, and then put your egg white halves on the plate.
2. Add your sweetener, cinnamon and mayonnaise to your yolks, mashing them together.
3. Transfer the yolk mixture to your white halves before serving.

Chocolate & Strawberry Smoothie

Serves: 1

Time: 5 Minutes

Calories: 273

Protein: 24 Grams

Fiber: 1 Grams

Fat: 17 Grams

Net Carbs: 3 Grams

Ingredients:

- 3 Strawberries, Frozen
- 1 Cup Water
- 3 Tablespoons Heavy Whipping Cream
- 1/3 Chocolate Whey protein Powder, Low Carb

Directions:

1. Blend all ingredients until smooth.

Frozen Coffee

Serves: 1

Time: 5 Minutes

Calories: 488

Protein: 3 Grams

Fiber: 0 Grams

Fat: 32 Grams

Net Carbs: 0 Grams

Ingredients:

- 7-10 Ice Cubes
- ½ Cup Whipped Cream
- 1 Cup Coffee, Cold Brew
- 1/3 Cup Heavy Whipping Cream
- 2 Tablespoons Vanilla Bean Sweetener, Sugar Free

Directions:

1. Place all of your ingredients except for your whipped cream into a blender, blending until smooth.
2. Top with whipped cream.

Keto Porridge

Serves: 1

Time: 15 Minutes

Calories: 249

Protein: 17.82 Grams

Fiber: 14 Grams

Fats: 13.07 Grams

Net Carbs: 5.78 Grams

Ingredients:

- 2 Tablespoons Coconut Flour
- 2 Tablespoons Vanilla protein Powder
- 3 tablespoons Golden Flaxseed Meal
- 1 ½ Cups Almond Milk, Unsweetened
- Powdered Erythritol to Taste

Directions:

1. Start by mixing your flaxseed meal, protein powder and coconut flour together in a bowl.
2. Add your mixture to a saucepan before adding in your almond milk turn the heat to medium, and then allow it to thicken.
3. Add in your preferred amount of liquid sweetener, and then serve warm.

Macadamia & Salted Chocolate Smoothie

Serves: 1

Time: 5 Minutes

Calories: 165

Protein: 12 Grams

Fiber: 3 Grams

Fat: 2 Grams

Net Carbs: 1 Gram

Ingredients:

- 2 Tablespoons Macadamia Nuts, Salted
- 1/3 Cup Chocolate Whey Protein Powder, Low Carb
- 1 Cup Almond Milk, Unsweetened

Directions:

1. Blend everything until smooth.

Bacon & Cheddar Omelet

Serves: 1

Time: 20 Minutes

Calories: 386

Protein: 24.86 Grams

Fiber: 0 Grams

Fat: 20.25 Grams

Net Carbs: 1.86 Grams

Ingredients:

- 2 Eggs, Large
- 1 Ounce Cheddar Cheese
- 1 Teaspoon Chives, Chopped
- 1 Teaspoon Bacon Fat
- 2 Slices Bacon, Cooked

Directions:

1. Place a pan over medium-low, and then add in your bacon fat. Add your eggs, seasoning with your chives.
2. Once the edges of your eggs have set you can add your bacon to the center. Allow it to cook for about thirty seconds, and then turn on your burner. Add in your bacon and cheese, folding it over, and then serving warm.

Bacon & Eggs

Serves: 1

Time: 25 Minutes

Calories: 761

Protein: 32.77 Grams

Fiber: 0 Grams

Fat: 68.15 Grams

Net Carbs: 3.68

Ingredients:

- 1/3 Cup Heavy Whipping Cream
- 4 Slices Bacon
- 1 Tablespoon Butter
- Sea Salt to Taste
- 3 Eggs, Large & Room Temperature

Directions:

1. Start by heating your oven to 350, and then lay your bacon on a baking sheet. Cook for ten to fifteen minutes or until crispy.
2. Add your eggs to a bowl, whisking with your cream lightly.
3. Heat your pan to medium-low, and then add in your butter.
4. Once your butter is melted, add in your eggs, and allow them to set.
5. Make a figure eight pattern with your spatula when stirring lightly.
6. Remove your eggs once set, and serve with your bacon.

Eggs Benedict

Serves: 1

Time: 25 Minutes

Calories: 488

Protein: 25.8 Grams

Fiber: 2.1 Grams

Fat: 40.6 Grams

Net Carbs: 3.8 Grams

Ingredients:

- 3 Cups Spinach, Fresh
- 2 Eggs, Large
- 2 Slices Ham
- 1 Serving Hollandaise Sauce, Keto Friendly
- Sea Salt to Taste

Directions:

1. Start by balancing your spinach. To do this wash and pat dry your spinach leaves, and then bring a pot to boil using high heat. Fill a bowl with ice water, and then place your spinach in the boiling water. Allow it to cook for thirty to sixty seconds, and then transfer it to the ice water. Strain your spinach and remove it. Make sure that the leaves are squeezed out.
2. Poach your eggs, filling a saucepan with water and adding a dash of sea salt. Crack your egg into a cup, and when the water boils reduce the heat to low. Create a whirlpool in the water so the egg white wraps around the yolk as you place it in the water, lowing the cup an inch into the water to do so. Cook or three minutes.
3. Remove the egg, and then place it in a bowl full of cold water or about twenty seconds.
4. Transfer your eggs to a plate, and then put the cooked spinach on a serving plate. Top it with your ham and poached egg before serving.

Spanakopita

Serves: 2

Time: 30 Minutes

Calories: 366

Protein: 22.4 Grams

Fat: 28 Grams

Fiber: 5.4 Grams

Net Carbs: 4.5 Grams

Ingredients:

- 3 Ounces Feta Cheese, Crumbled
- 3 Ounces Spinach, Cooked & Drained
- 4 Tablespoons Flax Meal
- 1 Tablespoon Cream Cheese, Heaped
- ¾ Cup Mozzarella, Shredded

Directions:

1. Start by melting your cream cheese and mozzarella in the microwave for a minute, and then check it halfway through.
2. Once your dough is complete, then add in your flax meal, combining until it's mixed well.
3. Roll the dough in between parchment paper. Peel of the parchment paper, adding in the crumbled feta and drained spinach into the center
4. Fold it over, and seal the dough.
5. Poke holes into it to release steam, baking at 400 for fifteen to twenty minutes. It should be firm to the touch and look golden brown.
6. Remove from the oven, and allow to cool before slicing to serve.

Green Berry Smoothie

Serves: 2

Time: 10 Minutes

Calories: 436

Protein: 28 Grams

Fiber: 5 Grams

Fat: 36 Grams

Net Carbs: 6 Grams

Ingredients:

- 1 Scoop Vanilla Protein Powder
- 1 Tablespoon Coconut Oil
- ¾ Cup Cream Cheese
- ½ Cup Kale, Shredded
- ½ Cup Raspberries
- 1 Cup Water

Directions:

1. Blend everything together until smooth.

Cinnamon Smoothie

Serves: 2

Time: 5 Minutes

Calories: 492

Protein: 18 Grams

Fiber: 2 Grams

Fat: 47 Grams

Net Carbs: 6 Grams

Ingredients:

- 2 Cups Coconut Milk
- 1 Scoop Vanilla Protein Powder
- 1 Teaspoon Ground Cinnamon
- 5 Drops Liquid Sweetener
- ½ Teaspoon Vanilla Extract

Directions:

1. Blend everything together until smooth.

Breakfast Bake

Serves: 8

Time: 1 Hour

Calories: 303

Protein: 17 Grams

Fiber: 1 Gram

Fat: 24 Grams

Net Carbs: 3 Grams

Ingredients:

- 1 lb. Homemade Sausage
- 8 Eggs, Large
- 2 Cups Spaghetti Squash, Cooked
- 1 Tablespoon Oregano, Chopped & fresh
- ½ Cup Cheddar Cheese, Shredded

Directions:

1. Start by heating your oven to 375, and then grease a nine by thirteen casserole dish using olive oil.
2. Put a skillet that's oven proof over medium-high heat. Cook your sausage for about five minutes.
3. Whisk your eggs, oregano and squash together. Season if desired.
4. Cook your sausage and egg mixture until combined, pouring it into your casserole dish.
5. Sprinkle your casserole with cheese, covering loosely.
6. Bake for thirty minutes before removing the foil. Uncover, cooking for another fifteen minutes.
7. Allow it to stand for ten minutes before serving.

Peanut Butter Cup Smoothie

Serves: 2

Time: 5 Minutes

Calories: 486

Protein: 30 Grams

Fiber: 5 Grams

Fat: 40 Grams

Net Carbs: 6 Grams

Ingredients:

- 1 Cup Water
- ¾ Cup Coconut Cream
- 1 Scoop Chocolate Protein Powder
- 3 Ice Cubes
- 2 Tablespoons Peanut Butter, Natural

Directions:

1. Blend until smooth.

Pesto Scrambled Eggs

Serves: 1

Time: 10 Minutes

Calories: 467

Protein: 20.4 Grams

Fiber: 0.7 Grams

Fat: 41.5 Grams

Net Carbs: 2.6 Grams

Ingredients:

- 3 Eggs, Large
- 1 Tablespoon Pesto
- 1 Tablespoon Ghee
- 2 Tablespoons Creamed Coconut Milk
- Sea Salt to Taste

Directions:

1. Start by cracking your egg into a bowl, seasoning with salt and beating with a fork.
2. Pour your eggs into a pan, adding in your ghee. Turn the heat on low, stirring frequently.
3. Add your pesto in, continuing to stir.
4. Take your pan off of heat, adding in your creamed coconut milk. Mix well.
5. Serve as desired.

Chapter 2: Lunch Recipes

Basil & Tomato Soup

Serves: 4

Time: 20 Minutes

Calories: 239

Protein: 3 Grams

Fiber: 2 Grams

Fat: 22 Grams

Net Carbs: 7 Grams

Ingredients:

- 14.5 Ounces Tomatoes, Diced
- 2 Ounces Cream Cheese
- ¼ cup Heavy Whipping Cream
- ¼ Cup Basil, Fresh & Chopped
- 4 Tablespoons Butter

Directions:

1. Pour your tomatoes into a blender with their juices, pureeing until completely smooth.
2. Cook in a saucepan over medium heat, adding in your heavy cream, butter, and cream cheese. Cook or ten minutes while stirring frequently. It should be melted and combined.
3. Add in your basil, seasoning as desired. Continue to cook for five more minutes, stirring frequently.
4. Use an immersion blender to blend until smooth.
5. Serve immediately.

Caprese Salad

Serves: 2

Time: 15 Minutes

Calories: 451

Protein: 19.75 Grams

Fiber: 1.15 Grams

Fat: 39.46 Grams

Net Carbs: 4.34 Grams

Ingredients:

- 1 Tomato, Large
- 3 Tablespoons Olive Oil
- ¼ Cup Basil, Fresh & Chopped
- 6 Ounces Mozzarella Cheese
- Sea Salt to Taste

Directions:

1. Pulse your basil and two tablespoons of olive oil in your food processor. Slice your tomato into slices that are about a quarter inch thick. You should get at least six slices.
2. Cut your mozzarella into slices, and then assemble your salad by layering your tomato, mozzarella and topping with your basil paste.
3. Season with pepper as desired.

Garlic Monkey Bread

Serves: 3

Time: 30 Minutes

Calories: 194

Protein: 8 Grams

Fiber: 4.7 Grams

Fat: 14.23 Grams

Net Carbs: 5.73

Ingredients:

- 1 Teaspoon Garlic Powder
- ¾ Cup Mozzarella Cheese, Shredded
- 2 Baby Eggplants, Cubed
- 2 Tablespoons Butter, Melted
- 1 Tablespoon Basil, Fresh & Chopped

Directions:

1. Start by turning your oven to 375, and then combine your melted butter and garlic powder together.
2. Take three miniature Bundt pan, and then layer about seven to ten cubes of eggplant.
3. Sprinkle with mozzarella, and then drizzle with a teaspoon of your garlic and butter mixture. Continue to layer, and top with your garlic butter and cheese.
4. Cook for about twenty minutes.
5. Allow to cool for five minutes before serving.

Cheesy Mug Melt

Serves: 1

Time: 5 Minutes

Calories: 268

Protein: 22.4 Grams

Fiber: 0 Grams

Fat: 17.99 Grams

Net Carbs: 3.83 Grams

Ingredients:

- 2 Ounces Roast Beef Slices
- 1 ½ Tablespoons Green Chiles, Diced
- 1 ½ Ounces Pepper Jack Cheese, Shredded
- 1 Tablespoon Sour Cream

Directions:

1. Layer your roast beef on the bottom of your mug, breaking it into smaller pieces.
2. Add in a half a tablespoon of sour cream, then a half tablespoon of green Chile and a half an ounce of pepper jack cheese. Continue to layer until all of your ingredients are gone, and then microwave for one to two minutes.
3. Serve warm.

BLT Salad

Serves: 2

Time: 20 Minutes

Calories: 278

Protein: 15 Grams

Fiber: 3 Grams

Fat: 20 Grams

Net Carbs: 7 Grams

Ingredients:

- 4 Bacon Slices
- ½ Head Iceberg Lettuce, Halved
- 2 Tablespoons Blue Cheese Salad Dressing, Keto Friendly
- ¼ Cup Blue Cheese, Crumbled
- ½ Cup Grape Tomatoes, Halved

Directions:

1. Place a skillet over medium-high heat, cooking your bacon until crispy on both sides. This should take about eight minutes. Transfer it to a paper towel so that it can drain, allowing it to cool for five minutes. Chop your bacon.
2. Put your wedges on two places, topping with your other ingredients to serve.

Mug Lasagna

Serves: 1

Time: 5 Minutes

Calories: 318

Protein: 20.45 Grams

Fiber: 1.1 Grams

Fat: 23.54 Grams

Net Carbs: 5.39 Grams

Ingredients:

- 1/3 Zucchini
- 3 Ounces Mozzarella Cheese, Whole Milk
- 2 Tablespoons Ricotta, Whole Milk
- 3 Tablespoons Marinara, Keto Friendly

Directions:

1. Slice your zucchini thin, and then place them on the bottom of your mug. Add in a tablespoon of marinara, and then layer on your zucchini.
2. Spread a tablespoon of ricotta over it, and then add in more marinara. Continue to layer until you run out of ingredients, topping with mozzarella.
3. Microwave for three to four minutes, and then serve warm.

Roasted Brussel Sprout Salad

Serves: 2

Time: 25 Minutes

Calories: 287

Protein: 14 Grams

Fiber: 10 Grams

Fat: 19 Grams

Net Carbs: 13 Grams

Ingredients:

- ¼ Cup Parmesan Cheese, Grated
- ¼ Cup Hazelnuts, Whole & Skinless
- 1 Tablespoon Olive Oil
- 1 lb. Brussel Sprouts
- Sea Salt to Taste

Directions:

1. Start by heating your oven to 350. Line a baking sheet with parchment paper, and then trim the bottom of your Brussel sprouts.
2. Put your leaves in a medium bowl, and make sure they're broken apart.
3. Toss the leaves with your olive oil, seasoning with sea salt.
4. Spread the leaves on your baking sheet.
5. Roast for ten to fifteen minutes. They should be crisp and lightly browned.
6. Divide between bowls, and then toss all other ingredients together.
7. Serve immediately.

Green Spring Salad

Serves: 1

Time: 10 Minutes

Calories: 393

Protein: 13.87 Grams

Fiber: 1.83 Grams

Fat: 36.11 Grams

Net Carbs: 4.27 Grams

Ingredients:

- 2 Ounces Mixed Greens
- 2 Slices Bacon
- 2 Tablespoons Shaved Parmesan
- 2 Tablespoons Raspberry Vinaigrette, Keto Friendly
- 3 Tablespoons Roasted Pine Nuts

Directions:

1. Cook your bacon until crisp, and then crumble it.
2. Toss all of your ingredients together, serving with bacon and your vinaigrette.

Taco Soup

Serves: 4

Time: 4 Hours 10 Minutes

Calories: 422

Protein: 25 Grams

Fiber: 1 Grams

Fat: 33 Grams

Net Carbs: 5 Grams

Ingredients:

- 1 lb. Ground Beef
- 2 Cups Beef Broth
- 10 Ounces Diced Tomatoes, Canned
- 1 Tablespoon Taco Seasoning
- 8 Ounces Cream Cheese

Directions:

1. Preheat your slow cooker, and then take a skillet placing it over medium-high heat. Sauté your ground beef, browning it for eight minutes. Season if desired.
2. Add your beef broth, tomatoes, taco seasoning, ground beef and cream cheese into your slow cooker.
3. Cover, cooking on low for four hours. Make sure to stir occasionally, and serve warm.

Bacon Hot Dogs

Serves: 6

Time: 25 Minutes

Calories: 283

Protein: 13.63 Grams

Fiber: 0.05 Grams

Fat: 19.26 Grams

Net Carbs: 2.08 Grams

Ingredients:

- ½ Teaspoon Garlic Powder
- ½ Teaspoon Onion Powder
- 2 Ounces Cheddar Cheese
- 12 Slices Bacon
- 6 Beef Hot Dogs, Large

Directions:

1. Start by heating your oven to 400, and then slit your hot dogs. Insert a slice of cheese into it.
2. Wrap your hot dogs in two slices of bacon, securing the ends using toothpicks.
3. Place them on a cookie sheet, and then season them.
4. Bake for about forty minutes, serving warm.

Egg Drop Soup

Serves: 1

Time: 5 Minutes

Calories: 289

Protein: 15.3 Grams

Fiber: 0 Grams

Fat: 23.24 Grams

Net Carbs: 2.92 Grams

Ingredients:

- 1 Teaspoon Chili Garlic Paste
- 2 Eggs, Large
- ½ Cube Chicken Bouillon
- 1 Tablespoons Bacon Fat
- 1 ½ Cups Chicken Broth

Directions:

1. Place a pan over medium high heat, adding in your bouillon cube, chicken broth, and bacon fat to your pan.
2. Bring it to a boil, adding in your chili garlic paste, and then stir well. Turn of the stove.
3. Beat your eggs and then pour them in your broth.
4. Stir and let sit for a moment before serving.

Goat Cheese Salad

Serves: 2

Time: 20 Minutes

Calories: 645

Protein: 33.2 Grams

Fiber: 4 Grams

Fat: 54.2 Grams

Net Carbs: 5.8 Grams

Ingredients:

- 1 ½ Cups Hard Goat Cheese, Grated
- 4 Cups Spinach, Fresh
- 4 Strawberries to Garnish
- ½ Cup Flaked Almonds, Toasted
- 4 Tablespoons Raspberry Vinaigrette, Keto Friendly

Directions:

1. Start by heating your oven to 400 degrees, and then line a baking sheet using parchment paper. Cut it in half, and then grate your goat cheese onto each half. Try to form two circles.
2. Bake for about ten minutes, and then place it over a bowl, allowing it to cool in a bowl shape. Peel the cheese off.
3. Toss all ingredients together in your cheese bowl, serving immediately.

Avocado Salad

Serves: 2

Time: 20 Minutes

Calories: 699

Protein: 14.2 Grams

Fiber: 15.5 Grams

Fat: 65.6 Grams

Net Carbs: 6.7 Grams

Ingredients:

- 2 Smalls Heads Lettuce
- 2 Avocados, Large
- 2 Cups Spinach, Fresh
- 1 Spring Onion, Medium
- 4 Slices Bacon

Directions:

1. Chop your spinach, avocados and lettuce.
2. Mix everything together.

Broccoli & Cheese Soup

Serves: 4

Time: 25 Minutes

Calories: 383

Protein: 10 Grams

Fiber: 1 Gram

Fat: 37 Grams

Net Carbs: 3 Grams

Ingredients:

- 2 Tablespoons Butter
- 1 Cup Heavy Whipping Cream
- 1 Cup Broccoli Florets, Chopped Fine
- 1 Cup Vegetable Broth
- 1 Cup Sharp Cheddar Cheese, Shredded

Directions:

1. Place your butter in a saucepan, placing it over medium heat.
2. Add in your broccoli, cooking until tender which should take five minutes.
3. Add in your vegetable broth and cream, stirring constantly.
4. Season as desired, cooking for ten to fifteen minutes. Stir occasionally and allow your soup to thicken.
5. Turn the heat to low, and then add in your cheddar cheese.
6. Serve warm.

Chapter 3: Snack Recipes

Smoked Salmon Fat Bombs

Serves: 12

Time: 2 Hours 10 Minutes

Calories: 193

Protein: 8 Grams

Fiber: 0 Grams

Fat: 18 Grams

Net Carbs: 0 Grams

Ingredients:

- ½ Cup Goat Cheese, Room Temperature
- 2 Teaspoons Lemon Juice, Fresh
- ½ Cup Butter, Room Temperature
- 2 Ounces Smoked Salmon
- Black Pepper to Taste

Directions:

1. Start by putting parchment paper over a baking sheet, and then take out a medium bowl.
2. Stir your butter, goat cheese, smoked salmon, pepper and lemon juice together.
3. Scoop it into twelve mounds.
4. Refrigerate for two to three hours.
5. Store in your fridge for up to one week.

Bacon Smokies

Serves: 4

Time: 40 Minutes

Calories: 242.27

Protein: 14.25 Grams

Fiber: 0.37 Grams

Fat: 18.61 Grams

Net Carbs: 2.67 Grams

Ingredients:

- 24 Little Smokies (Sausages)
- 3 Tablespoons BBQ Sauce, Keto Friendly
- Sea Salt & Black Pepper to Taste
- 6 Slices Bacon

Directions:

1. Start by heating your oven to 375, and then cut your bacon into quarter pieces.
2. Put your sausages on each one, and then roll the bacon over them, inserting a toothpick to keep them together
3. Cook for twenty-five minutes, and then baste with BBQ sauce. Bake or another ten to twelve minutes.
4. Serve warm.

Pepper & Bacon Fat Bombs

Serves: 12

Time: 1 Hour 10 Minutes

Calories: 89

Protein: 3 Grams

Fiber: 0 Grams

Fat: 8 Grams

Net Carbs: 0 Grams

Ingredients:

- 2 Ounces Goat Cheese, Room Temperature
- 2 Ounces Cream Cheese, Room Temperature
- ¼ Cup Butter, Room Temperature
- 8 Bacon Slices, Chopped & Cooked
- Black Pepper to Taste

Directions:

1. Line a baking sheet with parchment paper, setting it to the side.
2. Stir all of your ingredients together, and then put them on your baking sheet.
3. Freeze for about an hour. You can store them in the fridge or two weeks.

Parmesan Chips

Serves: 8

Time: 15 Minutes

Calories: 133

Protein: 11 Grams

Fiber: 0 Grams

Fat: 11 Grams

Net Carbs: 1 Gram

Ingredients:

- 1 Teaspoon Butter
- 8 Ounces Parmesan Cheese, Full Fat & Shredded

Directions:

1. Start by heating your oven to 400.
2. Put parchment paper on a baking sheet, greasing it lightly with butter.
3. Spoon your parmesan into eight mounds spread evenly apart, and then flatten them.
4. Bake for five minutes. They should be brown around the edges, and then allow them to cool.
5. Store in the fridge for up to four days.

Burger Bacon Bombs

Serves: 12

Time: 1 Hour 10 Minutes

Calories: 249.17

Protein: 14.38 Grams

Fiber: 0 Grams

Fat: 20.31 Grams

Net Carbs: 1.37 Grams

Ingredients:

- 12 Slices of Bacon
- 12 Sausage Patties, Raw
- 12 Cubed Smoked Cheddar Cheese
- Cumin to Taste
- Onion Powder to Taste

Directions:

1. Start by heating your oven to 350, and then lay your sausage on a prepared cookie sheet.
2. Season your sausage patties, and then put a piece of cheese in the middle. Roll the sausage around the cheese to form a ball.
3. Wrap your sausage balls in bacon, and then bake for an hour.

Pesto Mushrooms

Serves: 5

Time: 20 Minutes

Calories: 409.6

Protein: 24.26 Grams

Fiber: 0.4 Grams

Fat: 33.21 Grams

Net Carbs: 2.8 Grams

Ingredients:

- 200 Grams Cremini Mushrooms
- 80 Grams Cream Cheese
- 25 Grams Basil Pesto
- 300 Grams Bacon

Directions:

1. Start by heating your oven to 375, and then combine your pesto and cream cheese together.
2. Lay your bacon slices on a cutting board, cutting them lengthwise in half.
3. Clean your mushrooms, removing the stalks.
4. Spoon your pesto into the caps, and then add in your cream cheese mixture.
5. Wrap your bacon around your mushrooms, baking for twenty to thirty minutes.
6. Serve warm or room temperature.

Pizza Fat Bombs

Serves: 6

Time: 10 Minutes

Calories: 101.33

Protein: 2.26 Grams

Fiber: 0.33 Grams

Fat: 9.62 Grams

Net Carbs: 1.69 Grams

Ingredients:

- 4 Ounces Cream Cheese
- 4 Slices Pepperoni
- 2 Tablespoons Sun Dried Tomato Pesto
- 2 Tablespoon Basil, Fresh & Chopped
- 8 Black Olives, Pitted

Directions:

1. Dice your olives and pepperoni, and then mix all ingredients together.
2. Form into balls, and garnish as desired.

Pimento Cheese Dip

Serves: 10

Time: 15 Minutes

Calories: 259.2

Protein: 6.32 Grams

Fiber: 0.02 Grams

Fat: 24.46 Grams

Net Carbs: 4.03 Grams

Ingredients:

- 1 Brick Cream Cheese
- 10 Cherry Peppers, Chopped
- 1 ½ Cups Cheddar Cheese, Shredded
- 1 Tablespoon Garlic, Minced
- Black Pepper to Taste

Directions:

1. Start by heating up your garlic in a pan over medium heat.
2. Drop your cream cheese in, allowing it to soften and stir occasionally.
3. Mix in your cheddar cheese, and then add in your chopped peppers.
4. Refrigerate until you're ready to serve.

Pork Bites

Serves: 3

Time: 1 Hour

Calories: 448

Protein: 19.61 Grams

Fiber: 0.2 Grams

Fat: 40.56 Grams

Net Carbs: 1.9 Grams

Ingredients:

- 10.5 Ounces Pork Belly Strips, Thin
- ¼ Onion, Large & Diced
- 1 Tablespoon Butter
- 1.76 Ounces Blue Cheese
- 4 Tablespoons Heavy Whipping Cream

Directions:

1. Turn your oven to a high baking setting, and then bake your pork belly in an oven safe dish. Season if desired. This should take thirty to forty-five minutes. They should turn a golden brown and be crispy.
2. Put your onion and butter in a pan, cooking it over medium heat. Caramelize your onions which should take about five minutes, and then add your cream.
3. Place your blue cheese in the pan once your cream is warm, allowing it to melt.
4. Place it on high heat or about two minutes, and then place it into a dish.
5. Allow your pork belly to cool before cutting it into bite size pieces.
6. Serve warm.

Kale Chips

Serves: 4

Time: 20 Minutes

Calories: 80.5

Protein: 1.82 Grams

Fiber: 0.9 Grams

Fat: 7.15 Grams

Net Carbs: 1.29 Grams

Ingredients:

- 1 Bunch Kale, Large
- 2 Tablespoons Olive Oil
- 1 Tablespoon Seasoned Salt

Directions:

1. Start by heating your oven to 350, and then remove your kale stems. Wash them and pat your kale dry.
2. Put your kale in a zipper top bag, and then add in your oil, shaking to coat.
3. Spread your kale on a prepared baking sheet, flattening the leaves.
4. Allow your kale to bake for twelve minutes, and then take them out of the oven.
5. Sprinkle with seasoned salt before allowing them to cool.

Spicy Tuna Deviled Eggs

Serves: 4

Time: 20 Minutes

Calories: 151

Protein: 10.7 Grams

Fiber: 0.2 Grams

Fat: 11.4 Grams

Net Carbs: 1.1 Grams

Ingredients:

- 4 Eggs, Large
- 3 Ounces Tuna, Drained
- 2 Tablespoons Mayonnaise
- 1 Tablespoon Sriracha Sauce
- 1 Spring Onion, Large & Sliced

Directions:

1. Put your eggs in a pot of water, and then bring it to a boil using high heat. Allow them to cook or thirteen minutes.
2. Transfer them to a bowl of ice water, allowing them to sit for five minutes.
3. Peel them, and then slice them in half. Remove the yolks, placing them in a bowl. Put your egg whites on a platter, and then add the rest of your ingredients to the bowl with the yolk.
4. Mash until combined well, and then place them back into your egg whites.
5. Garnish with more spring onions if desired.

Jalapeno Popper Deviled Eggs

Serves: 4

Time: 10 Minutes

Calories: 176

Protein: 10.2 Grams

Fiber: 0.1 Grams

Fat: 14.6 Grams

Net Carbs: 0.7 Grams

Ingredients:

- 4 Eggs, Large & Hardboiled
- 2 Tablespoons Mayonnaise
- 1/3 Cup Cheddar Cheese, Grated
- 2 Slices Bacon, Cooked & Crumbled
- 1 Jalapeno, Sliced

Directions:

1. Cut your eggs in half, removing the yolk and putting them in a bowl. Lay your egg whites on a platter.
2. Mix all of your remaining ingredients in with your yolks, mashing until they're well combined.
3. Put your egg yolk mixture back into your egg whites to serve.

Keto Pizza Bite

Yields: 21

Time: 20 Minutes

Calories: 61.29

Protein: 3 Grams

Fiber: 0 Grams

Fat: 5.3 Grams

Net Carbs: 0.16 Grams

Ingredients:

- 5.25 Ounces Mozzarella Cheese, Shredded
- 6 Ounces Pepperoni, Sliced

Directions:

1. Start by heating your oven to 400, and then take out two cookie sheets.
2. Place your pepperoni in our batches close together. Bake for five minutes. They should become crispy, and then sprinkle your cheese on top.
3. Bake it for another three minutes, and then lay them on a paper towel. This will help to drain away the excess grease.
4. Allow it to cool for about five minutes before serving.

Bacon Mozzarella Sticks

Serves: 3

Time: 1 Hour 25 Minutes

Calories: 260

Protein: 26 Grams

Fiber: 0 Grams

Fat: 18 Grams

Net Carbs: 0 Grams

Ingredients:

- 12 Bacon Strips, Uncured & Center Cut
- 6 Mozzarella Cheese Sticks, Whole Milk

Directions:

1. Take a baking sheet out and line it with parchment paper, putting your cheese ticks on the sheet. Freeze your cheese for an hour.
2. Heat your oven to 400, and then wrap the stick with two strips of bacon.
3. Bake them for fifteen minutes, serving warm.

Chicken Liver Bites

Serves: 4

Time: 15 Minutes

Calories: 309

Protein: 27.6 Grams

Fiber: 0.3 Grams

Fat: 21.1 Grams

Net Carbs: 1 Gram

Ingredients:

- 1 Teaspoon Paprika
- ½ Teaspoon Cayenne
- 1 Tablespoon Swerve
- 12 Slices Bacon
- 12 Pieces Chicken Liver

Directions:

1. Start by lining a baking sheet with foil and then preheat your oven broiler.
2. Sprinkle the chicken livers with seasoning if desired, and then wrap each one in a piece of bacon.
3. Mix your spices together, sprinkling both sides of your liver.
4. Broil for six to eight minutes, and then allow it to cool before serving.

Egg & Avocado Fat Bombs

Serves: 5

Time: 20 Minutes

Calories: 147

Protein: 2.2 Grams

Fiber: 1.4 Grams

Fat: 14.8 Grams

Net Carbs: 1.1 Grams

Ingredients:

- 2 Tablespoons Chives, Fresh & Chopped
- 1 Tablespoon Lemon Juice, Fresh
- ¼ Cup Mayonnaise
- ½ Avocado, Large
- 3 Egg Yolks, Large & Cooked

Directions:

1. Halve your avocados, removing the seed and peel.
2. Spoons your egg yolks into a bowl without breaking the whites.
3. Place your egg yolk and avocado into a food processor, blending with your lemon juice and mayonnaise. Process until smooth, and then place the mixture into your egg whites to serve.

Chocolate Dipped Bacon

Serves: 6

Time: 30 Minutes

Calories: 479

Protein: 30 Grams

Fiber: 1 Gram

Fat: 39 Grams

Net Carbs: 1 Gram

Ingredients:

- 1 lb. Bacon, Uncured & Center Cut
- 2 Tablespoons Golden Ghee
- 1 Ounce Chocolate, Unsweetened
- 1 Tablespoon Heavy Whipping Cream
- 1 Tablespoon Vanilla Bean Sweetener, Sugar Free

Serves:

1. Heat your oven to 400, and then line two baking sheets using parchment paper.
2. Lay the bacon strips in a single layer, and then cook them for fifteen minutes. Drain your bacon using paper towels.
3. Take out a microwave safe bowl, mixing your ghee and chocolate together. Microwave for fifteen second intervals, stirring each time, until it mixes together easily.
4. Add your heavy cream and sweetener in, mixing again until smooth.
5. Lay your bacon on a new sheet of parchment paper, drizzling your chocolate over one third of each slice, and then refrigerate or at least five minutes before serving.

Macadamia & Brazil Butter

Yields: 1 ¼ Cup

Time: 5 Minutes

Calories: 225

Protein: 2.8 Grams

Fiber: 2.7 Grams

Fat: 23.6 Grams

Net Carbs: 1.7 Grams

Ingredients:

- ½ Teaspoon Vanilla Powder
- ¼ Teaspoon Sea Salt, Fine
- 10 Brazil Nuts
- 2 Cups Macadamia Nuts

Directions:

1. Put all of your ingredients into a food processor, processing until smooth. You'll need to keep scraping the sides. This can take the full five minutes to get smooth.

Bacon & Egg Fat Bombs

Serves: 6

Time: 30 Minutes

Calories: 185

Protein: 5 Grams

Fiber: 0 Grams

Fat: 18.4 Grams

Net Carbs: 0.2 Grams

Ingredients:

- 2 Hardboiled Eggs, Large
- 2 Tablespoons Mayonnaise
- ¼ Cup Ghee
- 4 Slices Bacon, Large
- Sea Salt to Taste

Directions:

1. Start by heating your oven to 375, and then line a baking sheet with parchment paper. Lay your bacon out in strips, baking for ten to fifteen minutes. They should be crisp and golden brown
2. Cut your butter into pieces, and peel and quarter your eggs mash your butter and eggs together, adding in your mayonnaise and sea salt. Pour your bacon grease in, and then combine it. Set it in the fridge for twenty minutes.
3. Crumble your bacon, and then roll your egg mixture in it to form balls.

Salmon Mousse Rolls

Yields: 30

Time: 25 Minutes

Calories: 29

Protein: 1.6 Grams

Fiber: 0.2 Grams

Fat: 2.5 Grams

Net Carbs: 0.7 Grams

Ingredients:

- 8 Ounces Cream Cheese
- 1 Tablespoon Dill, Fresh + Some for Garnish
- 4 Ounces Smoked Salmon
- ½ Lemon, Juiced
- 2-3 Cucumbers

Directions:

1. Slice your cucumbers very thin and into long strips.
2. Place your dill, salmon, lemon and cream cheese in a blender, blending until smooth.
3. Spread your salmon mousse over the cucumber, and then roll it up tightly.
4. Serve chilled or room temperature.

Layered Fried Queso

Serves: 4

Time: 15 Minutes

Calories: 562

Protein: 29.55 Grams

Fiber: 4.4 Grams

Fat: 47.64 Grams

Net Carbs: 1.47 Grams

Ingredients:

- 5 Ounces Queso Blanco
- Red Pepper Flakes to Taste
- 2 Ounces Olives
- 1 ½ Tablespoons Olive Oil

Directions:

1. Make sure your cheese is chopped into cubes, and then heat your oil in a skillet using medium-high heat.
2. Add your cheese to the skillet, browning them on each side.
3. Press the cheese down with a spatula, and then flip it as necessary. Keep flipping to build layers, and then chop it after letting it stand for five minutes.
4. Serve warm or room temperature.

Cashew & Almond Butter

Yields: 1 Cup

Time: 20 Minutes

Calories: 205

Protein: 5.2 Grams

Fiber: 2.1 Grams

Fat: 19.4 Grams

Net Carbs: 3.4 Grams

Ingredients:

- 1 Cup Almonds, Blanched
- 1/3 Cup Cashew Nuts
- 4 Tablespoons Coconut Oil
- Sea Salt to Taste
- ½ Teaspoon Cinnamon

Directions:

1. Start by heating your oven to 350, and then bake for twelve to fifteen minutes.
2. Allow them to cool, and then process until smooth. You'll need to scrape the sides occasionally.
3. Add in your oil and continue to blend until smooth.

Coconut Chips

Serves: 4

Time: 10 Minutes

Calories: 259

Protein: 2.1 Grams

Fiber: 5.1 Grams

Fat: 26.2 Grams

Net Carbs: 2.5 Grams

Ingredients:

- 2 Cups Flaked Coconut, Desiccated
- 2 Tablespoons Coconut Oil, Melted
- ½ Teaspoon Vanilla Extract
- ½ Teaspoon Cinnamon
- 1 Tablespoon Swerve

Directions:

1. Start by heating your oven to 350, and then mix your coconut oil, vanilla, swerve and cinnamon in a bowl.
2. Pour the mixture over your flaked coconut, and then cook for four to seven minutes at 350 in your oven. Be careful that it doesn't overcook or it will become bitter.
3. Allow to cool before serving.

Jalapeno Poppers

Serves: 4

Time: 35 Minutes

Calories: 434

Protein: 24.2 Grams

Fiber: 1.2 Grams

Fat: 35.5 Grams

Net Carbs: 3.5 Grams

Ingredients:

- 12 Jalapeno Peppers, Deseeded
- 1 Cup Ricotta Cheese
- 12 Slices Bacon, Cut Lengthwise
- ½ Cup Gruyere Cheese, Grated
- 2 Tablespoons Cilantro, Fresh & Chopped

Directions:

1. Start by turning your oven to 400 degrees, and then wash your jalapenos before patting them dry.
2. Halve your jalapenos and deseed them.
3. Mix your Gruyere cheese, cilantro and ricotta together. Fill each jalapeno with the mixture.
4. Wrap your jalapenos in your bacon, baking for twenty to twenty-five minutes.

Caprese Skewers

Serves: 2

Time: 10 Minutes

Calories: 384

Protein: 24.5 Grams

Fiber: 3.1 Grams

Fat: 27.4 Grams

Net Carbs: 7.1 Grams

Ingredients:

- 2 Cups Cherry Tomatoes
- 2 Tablespoons Basil, fresh
- 2 Tablespoons Green Pesto
- 2 Cups Baby Mozzarella Cheese Balls
- ½ Cup Mixed Olives, Pitted

Directions:

1. Wash your basil and tomatoes, and then allow them to dry.
2. Mix your pesto and mozzarella together.
3. To assemble your skewers piece your mozzarella, olives and tomatoes together.
4. Garnish with basil before serving.

Butternut Squash Chips

Serves: 4

Time: 2 Hours

Calories: 104

Protein: 1 Gram

Fiber: 2.5 Grams

Fat: 6.9 Grams

Net Carbs: 9.9 Grams

Ingredients:

- 1 Butternut Squash
- 1 Teaspoon Gingerbread Spice Mix
- 2 Tablespoons Coconut Oil
- Sea Salt to Taste
- 3-6 Drops Liquid Sweetener

Directions:

1. Start by heating your oven to 250, and then peel your squash. Peel your squash into thin slices.
2. In a bowl mix your coconut oil, liquid sweetener and gingerbread spice together.
3. Place the mixture over your butternut squash, making sure it covers all of it.
4. Arrange your slices on a baking sheet that's been prepared with parchment paper. You'll need about two different sheets.
5. Place them in the oven, cooking for an hour and a half to two hour or until crispy.
6. Allow to cool before serving.

Salami Pinwheels

Serves: 2

Time: 6 Hours 20 Minutes

Calories: 583

Protein: 19 Grams

Fiber: 0 Grams

Fat: 54 Grams

Net Carbs: 7 Grams

Ingredients:

- 8 Ounces Cream Cheese, Room Temperature
- ¼ lb. Salami, Sliced Thin
- 2 Tablespoons Pepperoncini, Sliced

Directions:

1. Lay plastic wrap over your counter, putting your cream cheese in the center. Add another layer of plastic on top, and then use a rolling pin to roll it to about a quarter inch thick it should resemble a rectangle when you're done.
2. Put your salami slices on top of your cream cheese under the plastic wrap. Put a new player of plastic wrap on top of the salami, and then flip it over. Peel the cream cheese on this side, laying your pepperoncini on top of the exposed cream cheese.
3. Roll the layered ingredients into a tight log, and then allow it to chill or six hours.
4. Slice before serving.

Ramen Dip

Serves: 4

Time: 1 Hour 5 Minutes

Calories: 156

Protein: 3 Grams

Fiber: 0 Grams

Fat: 16 Grams

Net Carbs: 1 Gram

Ingredients:

- 6 Ounces Sour Cream
- 1 Chicken Ramen Seasoning Packet
- 2 Tablespoons Mayonnaise
- ¼ Cup Cream Cheese, Room Temperature

Directions:

1. Blend all ingredients together with a hand blender, and then refrigerate it for at least an hour before serving.

Bacon Jalapenos

Serves: 4

Time: 30 Minutes

Calories: 164

Protein: 9 Grams

Fiber: 0 Grams

Fat: 13 Grams

Net Carbs: 1 Gram

Ingredients:

- 10 Jalapenos
- 8 Ounces Cream Cheese, Room Temperature
- 1 lb. Bacon

Directions:

1. Start by heating your oven to 450, and then line a baking sheet using aluminum foil.
2. Halve your jalapenos, cleaning out the seeds and membranes.
3. Spoon some cream cheese into each jalapeno half, and then wrap each half with a slice of bacon, securing it with a toothpick.
4. Place your jalapenos on the baking sheet, baking for about twenty minutes.
5. Serve warm or room temperature.

Dill Deviled Eggs

Serves: 6

Time: 10 Minutes

Calories: 202

Protein: 14 Grams

Fiber: 0 Grams

Fat: 15 Grams

Net Carbs: 3 Grams

Ingredients:

- 12 Hardboiled Eggs, Large
- 6 Tablespoons Mayonnaise, Sugar Free
- 1 Tablespoon Dill, Dried
- 1 Teaspoon Sea Salt, Fine

Directions:

1. Slice your eggs in half lengthwise, separating the yolks from the whites. Place your yolks in a bowl, adding in the rest of your ingredients.
2. Mix until smooth, and then place the mixture back in your egg whites to serve.

Mozzarella Pizza

Serves: 2

Time: 20 Minutes

Calories: 324

Protein: 33 Grams

Fiber: 1 Gram

Fat: 20 Grams

Net Carbs: 3 Grams

Ingredients:

- 2 Cups Mozzarella Cheese, Shredded
- 1 Teaspoon Garlic Powder
- ½ Cup Tomato Sauce
- Parmesan Cheese, Grated
- 1 Teaspoon Pizza Seasoning, Divided

Directions:

1. Heat your oven to 400, and then line a baking sheet with parchment paper. You do not want to use aluminum foil.
2. Put your mozzarella on the sheet in a large rectangle, making sure that there aren't any holes. Sprinkle the garlic powder and just a pinch of your pizza seasoning all over the cheese. Bake it or twelve to fifteen minutes, and your cheese should be browned.
3. Allow it to cool on the baking sheet for three minutes.
4. Spread your tomato sauce on top of the cheese, and then sprinkle the parmesan over it. Add a little more pizza seasoning.
5. Place it back in the oven, cooking or another minute.
6. Serve warm.

Stuffed Portobello Mushrooms

Serves: 2

Time: 30 Minutes

Calories: 334

Protein: 14.3 Grams

Fiber: 2.3 Grams

Fat: 28.5 Grams

Net Carbs: 5.5 Grams

Ingredients:

- 4 Portobello Mushrooms
- 1 Cup Blue Cheese, Crumbled
- 2 Cups Lettuce
- 2 Tablespoons Olive Oil
- Fresh Thyme

Directions:

1. Start by turning your oven to 350, and then remove the stem.
2. Chop the stem pieces and add in your thyme.
3. Mix your blue cheese in with the thyme mixture, and then place the mixture into your mushroom caps. Bake for twenty to twenty-five minutes.
4. Serve drizzled with olive oil.

Orange Celeriac Chips

Serves: 4

Time: 50 Minutes

Calories: 112

Protein: 2.1 Grams

Fiber: 2.4 Grams

Fat: 7.6 Grams

Net Carbs: 7.7 Grams

Ingredients:

- 1 Teaspoon Paprika
- 2 Tablespoons Orange Juice, fresh
- 1 Celery Root, Large
- 2 Tablespoons Ghee
- 1 Tablespoon Orange Peel, finely Grated

Directions:

1. Start by heating the oven to 300, and then peel your celery. Slice your celery thin, and then pull out a small bowl.
2. In your bowl mix your orange peel, orange juice, ghee and paprika together.
3. Add in your celery, making sure it's completely coated.
4. Place them on a prepared baking sheet, and then cook or about thirty to forty minutes. They should be golden brown, and you'll need to check them every ten minutes to turn them as needed.

Sour Cream Pork Rinds

Serves: 4

Time: 2 Hours 40 Minutes

Calories: 278

Protein: 25 Grams

Fiber: 0 Grams

Fat: 19 Grams

Net Carbs: 1.5 Grams

Ingredients:

- 3 Tablespoons Sweet Cream Buttermilk Powder
- 1 Tablespoon Garlic Powder
- 2 Tablespoons Onion Powder
- 2 lbs. Pork Skin
- 3 Tablespoons Chives, Dried

Directions:

1. Line a baking sheet with parchment paper, and then cut the pork skin with kitchen shears. You should cut it into one inch pieces, and then put the skin side up on your baking sheet.
2. Bake it for two and a half hours, and then remove it from the oven.
3. In a bowl toss your pork rinds with all of your other ingredients before serving warm or at room temperature.

Eggplant Chips

Serves: 4

Time: 40 Minutes

Calories: 133

Protein: 1.3 Grams

Fiber: 4.3 Grams

Fat: 11.5 Grams

Net Carbs: 3.1 Grams

Ingredients:

- 2 Eggplants
- 3 Tablespoons Ghee
- 1 Garlic Clove, Minced
- 1 Tablespoon Rosemary, Fresh & Chopped
- Sea Salt to Taste

Directions:

1. Slice your eggplants thin, and then lay it on a prepared baking sheet in a single layer.
2. Sprinkle your eggplant with sea salt, and then allow or the water to leach out before baking. Use a paper towel to clean up the excess water.
3. Preheat your oven to 350, and then take out a small bowl. Melt your ghee, adding in your rosemary and garlic. Mix well.
4. Brush each side of your eggplant slices with the mixture, and then bake for twenty to thirty minutes or until crisp and golden brown.

Coconut & Pecan Nut Butter

Serves: 8

Time: 10 Minutes

Protein: 5 Grams

Fiber: 4.4 Grams

Fat: 11.6 Grams

Net Carbs: 2.1 Grams

Ingredients:

- ½ Teaspoon Cinnamon
- ½ Teaspoon Sea Salt, Fine
- 2 Cups Coconut, Unsweetened & Shredded
- 1 Cup Pecans
- 1 Teaspoon Vanilla Extract, Sugar Free

Directions:

1. Place your coconut and pecans into your food processor, processing until chopped.
2. Mix in your cinnamon and vanilla extract, pulsing or another thirty seconds to a minute. Make sure that you scrape the mixture from the sides and pulse more.
3. Continue to pulse until it's a smooth blend. This can take up to ten minutes.

Spicy Zucchini Chips

Serves: 4

Time: 1 Hour 30 Minutes

Calories: 54.4

Protein: 1.4 Grams

Fiber: 1.4 Grams

Fat: 3.8 Grams

Net Carbs: 3.2 Grams

Ingredients:

- 2 Zucchinis
- 1 Lime, Juiced
- 1 Tablespoon Lime Zest
- 1 Tablespoon Olive Oil
- 1 Teaspoon Chili Powder

Directions:

1. Start by heating your oven to 230, and then mix your lime juice, zest and chili pepper together in a bowl.
2. Thinly slice your zucchini, and then cover the slices with your spice mixture.
3. Prepare a baking sheet with parchment paper, and then lay them out in a single line. Cook for forty-five to sixty minutes or until crispy and golden.
4. Allow to cool before serving.

Mushrooms

Serves: 4

Time: 1 Hour 35 Minutes

Calories: 169

Protein: 3.2 Grams

Fiber: 2 Grams

Fat: 15.5 Grams

Net Carbs: 3.9 Grams

Ingredients:

- 10.6 Ounces Portobello Mushrooms
- 4 Tablespoons Ghee, Melted
- ½ Teaspoon Sea Salt, Fine
- Ground Black Pepper to Taste

Directions:

1. Start by turning your oven to 300, and then slice your mushrooms thin.
2. Line a baking sheet with parchment paper, and then place them in a single layer on your baking sheet.
3. Brush your sliced mushrooms down with your ghee, sprinkling them with sea salt and black pepper.
4. Bake them or forty-five to sixty minutes. You will need to turn the tray two to three times during this time. Your mushrooms should be golden brown and crisp.

Chapter 4: Dinner Recipes

Sausage Stuffed Zucchini

Serves: 4

Time: 45 Minutes

Calories: 388

Protein: 21.7 Grams

Fiber: 4.4 Grams

Fat: 29.8 Grams

Net Carbs: 7 Grams

Ingredients:

- 4 Round Zucchinis
- 2 Tablespoons Ghee
- ½ Chorizo Sausage
- 1 ½ Cups Wild Mushrooms
- 1 Cup Cheddar Cheese, Grated

Directions:

1. Heat your oven to 350, and then cut the tops off of your zucchini.
2. Use a melon baller to scoop the flesh out, leaving a shell that's a half inch thick. Put the flesh in a bowl.
3. Melt your ghee and brush your squash down with it, and then put it on a baking sheet for twenty minutes. It should be tender.
4. Dice your mushrooms and chorizo, and then use the remaining ghee in a pan over medium-high heat until its crisp. This should take about five minutes.
5. Add your mushrooms, cooking or another three to five minutes, making sure to stir it occasionally.

6. Add in the flesh from your zucchini, cooking for another three to five minutes. Grate your cheddar cheese, adding it to your mushroom mixture, mixing until it's well combined.
7. Season your zucchinis if desired, but spoon the mixture into your zucchini shells. Cook it for fifteen to twenty minutes.

Beef Ragu

Serves: 4

Time: 20 Minutes

Calories: 645

Protein: 37.8 Grams

Fiber: 2.6 Grams

Fat: 51.1 Grams

Net Carbs: 5.7 Grams

Ingredients:

- 1.8 lbs. Ground Beef
- ¼ Cup Red Pesto
- 1 Tablespoon Ghee
- 4 Tablespoons Parsley, Fresh & Chopped
- Sea Salt to Taste

Directions:

1. Grease a pan with ghee, and then brown your meat in a pan over medium heat. This should take five to eight minutes.
2. Add in your red pesto and parsley, cooking over medium heat for about five more minutes.
3. Serve warm. It's best served over zoodles.

Parmesan Salmon with Asparagus

Serves: 2

Time: 20 Minutes

Calories: 434

Protein: 42 Grams

Fiber: 5 Grams

Fat: 26 Grams

Net Carbs: 6 Grams

Ingredients:

- 2 Salmon Fillets, 6 Ounces Each & Skin On
- Sea Salt to Taste (Optional)
- 1 lb. Asparagus, Trimmed
- 2 Cloves Garlic, Minced
- 3 Tablespoons Butter
- ¼ Cup Parmesan Cheese, Grated

Directions:

1. Start by heating your oven to 40, lining a baking sheet with oil.
2. Take a paper towel and pat your salmon dry, and then season it as desired.
3. Put your salmon on your baking sheet, arranging the asparagus around it.
4. Place a pan over medium heat, melting your butter. Add in your garlic, cooking for about three minutes or until your garlic begins to brown.
5. Drizzle this sauce over your salmon and asparagus.
6. Sprinkle your salmon and asparagus with parmesan, baking for about twelve minutes. Your salmon should be cooked all the way through and laky, and your asparagus should be tender.
7. Serve warm.

Lemon Butter Cod

Serves: 2

Time: 30 Minutes

Calories: 284

Protein: 32 Grams

Fiber: 0 Grams

Fat: 18 Grams

Net Carbs: 1 Gram

Ingredients:

- 4 Tablespoons Salted Butter, Divided
- 4 Thyme Sprigs, Fresh & Divided
- 4 Teaspoons Lemon Juice, Fresh & Divided
- 4 Cold Fillets, 6 Ounces Each
- Sea Salt to Taste

Directions:

1. Start by heating your oven to 400.
2. Season your cold with sea salt on both side, and then take out four pieces of foil. Each piece of foil should be three times the size of your foil. Divide your butter, lemon juice and thyme among your our fillets, and then fold the foil to form a pouch so that your fillet is inside. Put these packets on your baking sheet.
3. Bake for twenty minutes, and then open the pouches carefully to allow the steam to get out before serving warm.

Sole Asiago

Serves: 4

Time: 20 Minutes

Calories: 406

Protein: 29 Grams

Fiber: 3 Grams

Fat: 31 Grams

Net Carbs: 3 Grams

Ingredients:

- 4 Sole Fillets, 4 Ounces
- 2 Eggs, Beaten
- ¾ Cup Almonds, Ground
- ¼ Cup Asiago Cheese
- 2 ½ Tablespoons Coconut Oil, Melted

Directions:

1. Start by heating your oven to 350, and then take a baking sheet and line it with parchment paper. Pat your fish down with a few paper towels.
2. Stir your almonds and cheese together.
3. Take out another bowl, beating your eggs in it.
4. Drag your sole through the egg and then press it into your almond mixture. Do this for all of your fillets, and then brush both sides of each piece down using your coconut oil.
5. Bake the fish until its cooked all the way through, which should take about eight minutes.
6. Serve warm.

Pork Belly

Serves: 4

Time: 2 Hours 15 Minutes

Calories: 806

Protein: 23.7 Grams

Fiber: 1 Grams

Fat: 81.6 Grams

Net Carbs: 2.6 Grams

Ingredients:

- 2.2 lbs. Pork Belly, Raw
- 1 Brown Onion, Large
- 1 Tablespoon Sea Salt, Fine
- 2 Tablespoons Olive Oil
- 1 Handful Sage, Fresh

Directions:

1. Bring a pot of water to a simmer, and then make slices in the skin of the pork. Make sure you don't cut into the flesh.
2. Put the belly skin side down in a steamer pot, steaming for fifteen minutes. This will help for the skin to open up, letting the fats soften.
3. Heat your oven to 375, and then remove the belly from your steamer basket. Put the skin side up on a roasting pan, patting it down with paper towels.
4. Rub your pork belly down with an oil of choice, making sure it gets into the slits.
5. Sprinkle it with sea salt, massaging it into the meat. Flip it skin side down on your tray, roasting for an hour.
6. Increase the temperature to 430, and then take it out of the oven.
7. Slice an onion into thick rounds, placing it in the bottom of your roasting tray along with your sage leaves.
8. Turn the meat over so that the skin side is up, placing it on top of your onions.

9. Put it back in the oven, roasting it for another half hour. The skin should turn bubbly and crisp.

Coconut Haddock

Serves: 4

Time: 25 Minutes

Calories: 299

Protein: 20 Grams

Fiber: 3 Grams

Fat: 24 Grams

Net Carbs: 1 Gram

Ingredients:

- 4 Haddock Fillets, Boneless & 5 Ounces
- 2 Tablespoons Coconut Oil, Melted
- 1 Cup Coconut, Shredded & Unsweetened
- ¼ Cup Hazelnuts, Ground
- Sea Salt to Taste

Directions:

1. Heat your oven to 400 degrees, and then line a baking sheet with parchment paper. Set it to the side.
2. Pat your fish fillets down with your paper towel, seasoning it with sea salt.
3. Stir your hazelnuts and shredded coconut together.
4. Drag your fish fillets through this mixture until each side is coated thickly. Put your fish on the baking sheet, and then brush it down with coconut oil.
5. Bake your haddock until it turns golden. The fish should flake easily with a fork, which will take about twelve minutes.
6. Serve warm.

Roasted Pork Loin with Mustard Sauce

Serves: 8

Time: 1 Hour 20 Minutes

Calories: 368

Protein: 25 Grams

Fiber: 0 Grams

Fat: 29 Grams

Net Carbs: 2 Grams

Ingredients:

- 2 lbs. Pork Loin Roast, Boneless
- 3 Tablespoons Grainy Mustard
- 3 Tablespoons Olive Oil
- 1 ½ Cups Heavy Whipping Cream
- Sea Salt to Taste

Directions:

1. Start by turning your oven to 375, and then season your pork roast with your sea salt.
2. Brown your roast in a skillet on all sides. It should take about six minutes in total. Place it in a baking dish, and then bake for an hour.
3. Fifteen minutes before your roast is done, put a saucepan over medium heat, adding your heavy cream and mustard together.
4. Stir the sauce as you bring it to a simmer, and then turn the heat to low simmer your sauce until it becomes thick, which should take about five minutes. Put your sauce to the side.
5. Allow your pork to rest for ten minutes before you slice and serve it with your sauce drizzled over it.

Cajun Snow Crab

Serves: 2

Time: 15 Minutes

Calories: 643

Protein: 41 Grams

Fiber: 1 Gram

Fat: 51 Grams

Net Carbs: 3 Grams

Ingredients:

- 1 Lemon, Fresh & Quartered
- 3 Tablespoons Cajun Seasoning
- 2 Bay Leaves
- 4 Snow crab Legs, Precooked & Defrosted
- Golden Ghee

Directions:

1. Take out a large pot and fill it halfway with salted water, bringing it to a boil using high heat. Squeeze your lemon juice into the pot, and then toss in the remaining quarters. Add in your bay leaves and Cajun seasoning, letting it season your water for a full minute.
2. Add in your crab legs, making sure that they're submerged. Boil them for five to eight minutes with them submerged the entire time.
3. Melt your ghee, and serve it as a dipping sauce for your crab.

Barbacoa Beef Roast

Serves: 2

Time: 8 Hours 10 Minutes

Calories: 723

Protein: 66 Grams

Fiber: 5 Grams

Fat: 46 Grams

Net Carbs: 2 Grams

Ingredients:

- ½ Cup Beef Broth
- 1 lb. Beef Chuck Roast
- 4 Chipotle Peppers in Adobo Sauce
- 5 Ounces Green Jalapeno Chiles, Canned
- 2 Tablespoons Apple Cider Vinegar

Directions:

1. Start by turning your crockpot to low, and then season your chuck roast as desired before placing it into the crockpot.
2. Take a blender and blend your chipotle peppers in the adobo sauce, jalapenos, and apple cider vinegar. Pulse until it's a smooth consistency, and then add in your beef broth. Pulse a little more, and then pour it over the roast.
3. Cover your crockpot, cooking on low or eight hours.
4. Shred the meat before serving.

Bacon & Scallops

Serves: 4

Time: 40 Minutes

Calories: 550

Protein: 66 Grams

Fiber: 0 Grams

Fat: 27 Grams

Net Carbs: 7 Grams

Ingredients:

- 1 lb. Bacon, Uncured
- 2 lbs. Sea Scallops, Fresh & Patted Dry
- Lemon Wedges
- 3 Tablespoons Golden Ghee
- ¼ Cup Dry White Wine

Directions:

1. Line two baking sheets with parchment paper, turning your oven to 400.
2. Put your bacon strips on the sheet evenly, baking them for fifteen to twenty minutes or until crispy. Crumble it once it's cooled.
3. Pour the grease into a skillet, putting it over high heat.
4. Brown your scallops in the oil, cooking for three to our minutes on each side.
5. Set your scallops to the side, and then add your wine into the skillet. Use the wine to deglaze the pan, and then scrape the brown bits from the bottom. Add in your ghee to make your wine sauce.
6. Add in your scallops and bacons, tossing to coat them. Cook or another minute, and then serve warm.

Goat Cheese Burgers

Serves: 2

Time: 20 Minutes

Calories: 857

Protein: 48.9 Grams

Fiber: 1.4 Grams

Fat: 69 Grams

Net Carbs: 7.3 Grams

Ingredients:

- 14.1 Ounces Ground Beef
- 4.5 Ounces Goat Cheese
- 2 Tablespoons Ghee + More
- 1 Yellow Onion, Large & Sliced
- 1 Tablespoon Brown Sugar Substitute
- Sea Salt (Optional)

Directions:

1. Put your goat cheese in the freezer for a half hour, and then start to peel and slice your onion.
2. Take a pan, greasing it with two tablespoons f ghee, adding in your onion.
3. Use medium-low heat, and cook your onion for fifteen to twenty minutes. You'll need to stir occasionally, and they should caramelize.
4. Add in the brown sugar substitute, making sure it's incorporated. Allow the mixture to cook for another five minutes while stirring to keep it from burning. Set it to the side.
5. Heat your oven to 400, removing your cheese from the freezer, and then make two patties out of your ground beef.
6. Add the cheese in the middle, wrapping the patty around it. The cheese needs to be covered so it doesn't ooze out when you're cooking the burger.

7. Take an ovenproof skillet and grease it with your ghee, adding in your burgers. Season them with salt if you're using it, and then cook on high for a minute per side.
8. Transfer your skillet to the oven, baking for another seven to eight minutes.
9. Allow the burgers to rest for five minutes, and then top with your caramelized onions before serving.

Lamb Chops

Serves: 2

Time: 45 Minutes

Calories: 566

Protein: 47 Grams

Fiber: 2 Grams

Fat: 40 Grams

Net Carbs: 2 Grams

Ingredients:

- ¼ Cup Olive Oil
- ¼ Cup Mint, Fresh & Chopped
- 8 Lamb Rib Chops
- 1 Tablespoon Garlic, Minced
- 1 Tablespoon Rosemary, Fresh & Chopped

Directions:

1. Combine your mint, rosemary, garlic, and olive oil together in a bowl. Set a tablespoon of this mixture to the side.
2. Toss the lamb chops in the marinade, allowing them to marinate for a half hour.
3. Take a cast iron skillet, cooking your lamb over medium-high heat. It should be two minutes on each side for medium-rare.
4. Allow your lamb to rest for a few minutes, and then drizzle them with the remaining marinade before serving.

Pepper & Sausage Ragout

Serves: 4

Time: 45 Minutes

Calories: 422

Protein: 23 Grams

Fiber: 1 Gram

Fat: 34 Grams

Net Carbs: 4 Grams

Ingredients:

- 1 Cup Green Bell Pepper, Chopped
- 1 lb. Sausage
- 2 Cups Marinara Sauce

Directions:

1. Start by putting a saucepan over medium heat, adding in your marinara. Bring it to a simmer.
2. In another skillet, brown your sausage over medium heat. Break up any clumps, which will take about five minutes to make sure it's cooked all the way through. Take a slotted spoon and add your sausage to your marinara.
3. Add in the green bell pepper to your skillet, using the fat that was rendered from the sausage to cook it. Allow it to soften, which should take about three minutes. Add this to the marinara as well.
4. Cover the marinara, reducing the heat to low, and then allow it to simmer for a half hour.
5. Serve warm.

Chicken Quesadilla

Serves: 2

Time: 50 Minutes

Calories: 619

Protein: 79 Grams

Fiber: 0 Grams

Fat: 35 Grams

Net Carbs: 2 Grams

Ingredients:

- ¼ Cup Ranch Dressing
- ½ Cup Cheddar Cheese, Shredded
- 20 Slices Bacon, Center Cut
- 2 Cups Grilled Chicken, Sliced

Directions:

1. Start by heating your oven to 400, and then line a baking sheet using parchment paper. Weave your bacon into two rectangles. Bake your bacon for a half hour.
2. Lay the grilled chicken over your bacon square, drizzling it with ranch dressing, sprinkling it with cheddar cheese. Top it with the second bacon square, and then bake it for five to ten minutes.
3. Slice it to serve.

Chicken Skewers & Peanut Sauce

Serves: 2

Time: 1 Hour 25 Minutes

Calories: 586

Protein: 75 Grams

Fiber: 1 Gram

Fat: 29 Grams

Net Carbs: 5 Grams

Ingredients:

- 1 lb. Chicken Breast, Skinless & Chopped into Chunks
- 3 Tablespoons Soy Sauce, Divided
- ½ Teaspoon Sriracha Sauce + ¼ Teaspoon
- 3 Teaspoons Toasted Sesame Oil, Divided
- 2 Tablespoons Peanut Butter
- Sea Salt (Optional)

Directions:

1. Soak your skewers in water or about a half hour before you use them.
2. Heat your grill to low, making sure to oil it.
3. Thread your chicken through the skewers, and then cook or ten to fifteen minutes. You'll need to flip it halfway through.
4. While it cooks mix your Sriracha sauce, sesame oil, peanut butter and soy sauce together to make your peanut butter. Season with salt if you're using it, and then serve your chicken with this sauce for dipping.

Bacon Cups

Serves: 2

Time: 30 Minutes

Calories: 354

Protein: 19.5 Grams

Fiber: 3.5 Grams

Fat: 28 Grams

Net Carbs: 3 Grams

Ingredients:

- 2 Tablespoons Sour Cream
- 12 Bacon Slices
- ½ Avocado, Diced
- ¼ Head Romaine Lettuce, Chopped
- ½ Cup Grape Tomatoes, Halved

Directions:

1. Start by heating your oven to 400.
2. Take out a muffin tin, turning it upside down. Make a cross with two bacon strips halves, and then layer it with two more bacon strips half. This will make a circle, and you can use a toothpick to hold them together tightly. Repeat this with three more cups.
3. Bake your bacon over your muffin tin for twenty minutes. The bacon should be crisp, and then you can let them cool for ten minutes on a cooling rack.
4. Once they're firm, remove them from the muffin tins, filling each with your avocado, tomatoes, romaine lettuce, and sour cream before serving.

Mississippi Pot Roast

Serves: 4

Time: 8 Hours 5 Minutes

Calories: 504

Protein: 36 Grams

Fiber: 0 Grams

Fat: 34 Grams

Net Carbs: 6 Grams

Ingredients:

- 1 Ounce Dry Ranch Seasoning Packet
- 1 Ounce Au Jus Gravy Mix
- 8 Tablespoons Butter
- 1 Cup Pepperoncini, Whole
- 1 lb. Beef Chuck Roast

Directions:

1. Start by heating your crockpot to low, and then season your chuck roast if desired.
2. Sprinkle the ranch dressing and gravy mixture over your roast, and then put the butter on top of your roast in your crockpot, adding your pepperoncini around it.
3. Cover the crockpot, cooking for eight hours.
4. Shred the beef before serving.

Miso Salmon

Serves: 4

Time: 30 Minutes

Protein: 28.38 Grams

Fiber: 0.25 Grams

Fat: 9.23 Grams

Net Carbs: 0.78 Grams

Ingredients:

- 1 ¼ lb. Salmon Fillets with Skin
- Sea Salt to Taste
- 3 Tablespoons Sake
- 3 Tablespoons White Miso
- 2 Tablespoons White Wine

Directions:

1. Start by cut the salmon into fillets, and then season with your se salt. Allow it to sit for a half hour, and then take a tablespoon of sake and wet a paper towel with it. Dab the salt off of the fish.
2. Mix two tablespoons of your white wine, all of your miso and two tablespoons of sake into a bowl, and then pour a third of the marinade in a container. Put your fillets into it, and then allow it to refrigerate for at least a half an hour.
3. Heat your oven to 400, and then scrape the marinade of your fish.
4. Line a baking sheet with parchment paper, and then bake your salmon for twenty-five minutes.

Beef Wellington

Serves: 4

Time: 40 Minutes

Calories: 307.5

Protein: 23.6 Grams

Fiber: 1.5 Grams

Fat: 22.66 Grams

Net Carbs: 2.31 Grams

Ingredients:

- 2 Tenderloin Steaks, Halved
- 1 Tablespoon Butter
- 1 Cup Mozzarella Cheese, Shredded
- ½ Cup Almond Flour
- 4 Tablespoons Liver Pate

Directions:

1. Season your steaks if desired, and then put a pan over medium-high heat. Place your butter in the pan, allowing it to melt.
2. Once it starts to bubble, then cook your steak, turning it every two to three minutes. Make sure that each side is seared.
3. Heat your mozzarella for a minute in the microwave, and then stir in your flour. This will form a dough, and then put our dough on a slice of parchment paper.
4. Put another piece of parchment paper on top, and then roll it lat. Put a tablespoon of pate on our dough, and then cut the dough so that you can form a ball around your meat with the pate on the inside. Do this or all slices of the steak.
5. Turn your oven to 400, and then cook for twenty to thirty minutes. It should be a golden brown.

Chicken Roulades with Gruyere

Serves: 4

Time: 45 Minutes

Calories: 315

Protein: 42 Grams

Fiber: 1 Gram

Fat: 14 Grams

Net Carbs: 2 Grams

Ingredients:

- 3 Ounces Gruyere Cheese, Grated Fine
- 1 Onion, Diced
- 1 Tablespoon White Wine Vinegar
- 2 Chicken Breasts
- 2 Tablespoons + 1 Tablespoon Sage, Fresh & Chopped Fine (Optional)

Directions:

1. Start by heating your oven to 375, and then line a baking pan prepared with parchment paper. It's best to use an 11x13 inch pan.
2. Cut your chicken breasts with a butterfly cut, and then lay it flat.
3. Put each chicken breasts between two pieces of plastic wrap, and then tenderize it with a mallet. It should be about a quarter inch thick when you're done, and then season if desired. Seasoning is not needed.
4. Heat a skillet over medium heat, melting your button.
5. When the butter stops foaming, add in your onions, cooking over medium-low heat. Stir frequently while they caramelize.
6. Add in your white wine, scraping up any browned bits, and then add your vinegar when you have a syrupy texture. Add two tablespoons of your sage if you're using it, stirring until it's combined.
7. Lay your pieces out flat and then cut three pieces of twine. Put the filling over them, keeping them away from the edges. Sprinkle two ounces of your cheese on each breast, and you should have an ounce saved for later.
8. Roll each breast up before securing it with the twine.

9. Put them in your pan, and then sprinkle it with the remaining cheese and sage if you're using it.
10. Bake for thirty-five minutes.
11. Allow it to cool for five minutes before slicing.

Baked Chicken Wings

Serves: 5

Time: 50 Minutes

Calories: 773.2

Protein: 64.8 Grams

Fiber: 0 Grams

Fat: 57.09 Grams

Net Carbs: 0.52 Grams

Ingredients:

- 20 Pieces Chicken Drumsticks & Wings
- ¼ Cup Butter
- 2 Teaspoons Baking Powder
- 1 Teaspoon Baking Soda
- 1 Tablespoon Sea Salt, Fine

Directions:

1. Put all of your chicken into a plastic bag with your baking powder, sea salt and baking soda. Shake well, and then put them on a wire rack in the fridge. Leave them overnight.
2. Heat your oven to 450, and then bake for twenty minutes.
3. Flip your chicken, baking for another fifteen minutes. They should be crispy.
4. Toss with butter before serving.

Perfect Ribeye Steak

Serves: 3

Time: 20 Minutes

Calories: 430

Protein: 30.8 Grams

Fiber: 0 Grams

Fats: 31.7 Grams

Net Carbs: 0 Grams

Ingredients:

- 2 Ribeye Steaks (about 1.2 lbs.)
- Sea Salt & Black Pepper to Taste
- 3 Tablespoons Bacon Fat

Directions:

1. Start by heating your oven to 250, and then put your steaks on a wire rack, placing the wire wrap on top of the cookie sheet. Season it with your salt and pepper on all sides. You'll want to season heavily.
2. Bake until it reaches an internal temperature of 123.
3. Put your bacon grease in a skillet, and then wait until it's hot to put your steaks in. sear it for about forty-five seconds on each side.

Perfect Ribeye

Serves: 2

Time: 30 Minutes

Calories: 749.5

Protein: 38 Grams

Fiber: 0 Grams

Fat: 66 Grams

Net Carbs: 0 Grams

Ingredients:

- 16 Ounce Ribeye Steak
- 1 Tablespoon Duck at
- 1 Tablespoon Butter
- ½ Teaspoon Thyme, Fresh & Chopped
- Sea Salt to Taste

Directions:

1. Start by turning your oven to 400, and then take out a cast iron skillet. Place the skillet in your onion, and then start prepping your steak. Season it with oil and your sea salt.
2. Take your pan out of the oven, and then place it over medium heat. Add oil, and then sear your steak for about two minutes on each side
3. Flip your steak, cooking it in the oven or four to six minutes. Take your steak out, and then put it on low heat on the stove, putting your thyme and butter in the pan. Baste your steak for two to four minutes.
4. Allow it to sit for five minutes before serving.

Slow Roasted Pork Shoulder

Serves: 20

Time: 50 Minutes

Calories: 461

Protein: 30.3 Grams

Fiber: 0.1 Grams

Fat: 36.7 Grams

Net Carbs: 0.2 Grams

Ingredients:

- 8 lbs. Pork Shoulder
- 3 ½ Tablespoons Sea Salt, Fine
- 1 Teaspoon Onion Powder
- 1 Teaspoon Garlic Powder
- 2 Teaspoons Oregano

Directions:

1. Wash your pork before patting it dry, and then allow it to come to room temperature. This can take a few hours, and then turn the oven to 250. Rub it down with all of your spices.
2. Put your wire rack on a baking sheet, placing your pork shoulder on it and covering it with foil.
3. Bake your pork shoulder or eight to ten minutes. The internal temperature should be 190 degrees.
4. Remove the meat from your oven, covering the foil. Allow it to rest for fifteen minutes, and then heat it to 500 degrees.
5. Remove the foil, roasting it for twenty more minutes. Rotate it every five minutes.
6. Allow it to rest for about fifteen minutes before serving.

Spicy Blackberry Chicken Wings

Serves: 4

Time: 1 Hour 10 Minutes

Calories: 502.7

Protein: 34.5 Grams

Fiber: 2.3 Grams

Fat: 39.1 Grams

Net Carbs: 1.8 Grams

Ingredients:

- 3 lbs. Chicken Wings (about 20 pieces)
- ½ Cup Blackberry Chipotle Jam
- Sea Salt & Black Pepper to Taste
- ½ Cup Water

Directions:

1. Start by combining your water and jam together in a bowl, and this will make your marinade.
2. Place your chicken wings in a zipper top bag with two thirds of your marinade, and then season with sea salt and pepper. Allow it to marinate for at least thirty minutes or overnight depending on your preference.
3. Heat your oven to 400, getting out a baking sheet and wire wrap. Bake your chicken wings on top of the wire rack for fifteen minutes.
4. Brush the rest of your marinade over them, and then bake for another twenty to thirty minutes.

Harissa Chicken Skewers

Serves: 4

Time: 2 Hours

Calories: 389

Protein: 32.7 Grams

Fiber: 1.5 Grams

Fat: 26.8 Grams

Net Carbs: 2.4 Grams

Ingredients:

- 1.3 lbs. Chicken Breasts
- 1/3 Cup Harissa Paste
- 2 Tablespoons + 4 Tablespoons Olive Oil

Directions:

1. Start by cutting your chicken into one inch pieces.
2. In a bowl add your olive oil and harissa paste together.
3. Mix this paste into your chicken, and then allow it to marinate for one to two minutes.
4. Assemble the skewers, and then heat your oven to 440.
5. Cook for twelve to fifteen minutes. Your chicken should be browned and cook all the way through.

Beef & Broccoli Roast

Serves: 2

Time: 4 Hours 40 Minutes

Calories: 806

Protein: 74 Grams

Fiber: 6 Grams

Fat: 49 Grams

Net Carbs: 12 Grams

Ingredients:

- ½ Cup Beef Broth + More as Needed
- 1 Teaspoon Toasted Sesame Oil
- ¼ Cup Soy Sauce
- 16 Ounces Broccoli, Frozen
- 1 lb. Beef Chuck Roast

Directions:

1. Start by preheating your crockpot to low, and then season your chuck roast as desired before slicing it thin. Place your sliced beef into the crockpot.
2. In a bowl mix your beef broth, soy sauce, and sesame oil together. Make sure to mix it well before pouring it over the beef.
3. Cover your crockpot, cooking it for four hours before adding in the frozen broccoli.
4. Cook for another half hour, and add beef broth as needed.
5. Serve warm.

Kalua Pork & Cabbage

Serves: 2

Time: 8 Hours 10 Minutes

Calories: 550

Protein: 39 Grams

Fiber: 5 Grams

Fat: 41 Grams

Net Carbs: 5 Grams

Ingredients:

- 1 lb. Pork Butt Roast, Boneless
- 1 Tablespoon Smoked Paprika
- ½ Cup Water
- ½ Head Cabbage, Chopped
- Sea Salt to Taste

Directions:

1. Start by turning your crockpot to low, and then season your pork roast with your smoked paprika, sea salt and black pepper.
2. Put your roast in your crockpot before adding in your water.
3. Cover your crockpot, allowing it to cook on low for seven hours.
4. Take your pork roast out of the crockpot putting it on a plate.
5. Chop your cabbage and place it at the bottom of your crockpot before putting your pork roast back on top.
6. Cover your crockpot again, cooking for another hour.
7. Take your pork roast out of the crockpot once more, shredding it.
8. Serve your shredded pork over your cooked cabbage while it's still warm

Perfect Roast

Serves: 8

Time: 5 Hours 40 Minutes

Calories: 681

Protein: 90 Grams

Fiber: 0 Grams

Fat: 46.6 Grams

Net Carbs: 0.3 Grams

Ingredients:

- 5 lbs. Beef Rib Roast
- 1 Teaspoon Garlic Powder
- 1 Teaspoon Black Pepper
- 2 Teaspoons Sea Salt, Fine

Directions:

1. Start by letting your roast sit at room temperature for an hour.
2. Heat your oven to 357, combining all of your spices together.
3. Put your roast on a roasting rack, and then rub it down with spices.
4. Roast it for an hour, and then turn of the oven. Don't open the door. Allow the roast to sit in the oven for three hours. Thirty minutes before you serve, turn it back to 357, and then allow it to rest for ten minutes before serving.

Baked Pesto Seabass

Serves: 2

Time: 15 Minutes

Calories: 423

Protein: 29.3 Grams

Fiber: 0.7 Grams

Fat: 32.9 Grams

Net Carbs: 1.5 Grams

Ingredients:

- 4 Tablespoons Pesto
- 2 Sea Bass Fillets, Large
- 1 Tablespoon Ghee
- 1 Tablespoon Lemon Juice, Fresh
- Sea Salt to Taste

Directions:

1. Start by heating your oven to 400, and then put your fish skin side down on a baking sheet that's been prepared with parchment paper. Season with sea salt, brushing it down with your ghee. Squeeze your lemon juice over your sea bass.
2. Cook it in the oven to fen minutes, and then brush it down with your pesto.
3. Bake your seabass for another three to five minutes in the oven before serving.

Herb & Butter Pork Chops

Serves: 2

Time: 30 Minutes

Calories: 333

Protein: 31 Grams

Fiber: 0 Grams

Fat: 23 Grams

Net Carbs: 0 Grams

Ingredients:

- Sea Salt (Optional)
- 1 Tablespoon Butter + Some for Coating
- 2 Pork Chops, Boneless
- 1 Tablespoon Italian Seasoning
- 1 Tablespoon Olive Oil
- 1 Tablespoon Parsley, Fresh & Chopped

Directions:

1. Start by heating your oven to 350, and then coat your baking sheet with butter.
2. Pat your pork chops dry using a paper towel before placing them on your prepared baking dish. Season with salt and Italian seasoning.
3. Add your fresh parsley on top, and then drizzle your olive oil over the meat.
4. Top each pork chop with a half a tablespoon of butter.
5. Place them in the oven, baking for twenty to twenty-five minutes. Remember that thinner pork chops will cook faster than thicker ones, so make sure that you pay attention.
6. Serve warm.

Cheddar & Bacon Delight

Serves: 5

Time: 1 Hour 45 Minutes

Calories: 415.2

Proteins: 25.97 Grams

Fiber: 0.66 Grams

Fat: 32.44 Grams

Net Carbs: 2.69 Grams

Ingredients:

- 30 Bacon Slices
- 2 Tablespoons Chipotle Seasoning
- 2 Teaspoons Mrs. Dash Table Seasoning
- 5 Cups Spinach, Raw
- 2 ½ Cups Cheddar Cheese, Shredded

Directions:

1. Heat your oven to 375, and then weave your bacon together.
2. Season your bacon with the seasoning mixture. Add your cheese, leaving about an inch and half on each side. Add in your spinach, compressing it before you roll the bacon up. Make sure that it stays tight when you wrap it, and then season the outside.
3. Cover a baking sheet in foil, and then put it on a cooling rack on the baking sheet.
4. Bake your bacon wrap for sixty to seventy minutes, and do not open the oven door. It should have a crispy top once finished, and then allow it to cool for fifteen minutes before taking it off of the rack.
5. Allow it to cool slightly before slicing to serve.

Bacon Cordon Blue

Serves: 4

Time: 1 Hour 15 Minutes

Calories: 294.75

Protein: 37.69 Grams

Fiber: 0 Grams

Fat: 14.68 Grams

Net Carbs: 0.64 Grams

Ingredients:

- 8 Bacon Slices
- 4 Slices Black Forest Ham
- 2 Ounces Blue Cheese
- 2 Chicken Breasts, Boneless & Skinless

Directions:

1. Trim your breast up, and then separate the halves. Carefully slice them lengthwise to portion them. Lay it open, and then lay a piece of ham on each chicken breasts. Put your cheese in the middle, and then old the ham over your cheese, and then fold a third over to close.
2. Your chicken should be folded to cover your ham, and then take a slice of bacon, stretching it to wrap your chicken.
3. Use a second piece of bacon and wrap it end to end, and then secure your bacon with toothpicks.
4. Take out a skillet that's ovenproof, placing your chicken in it, and make sure your skillet has been greased.
5. Heat your oven to 325, and put the skillet over medium heat. Brown your bacon on all sides.
6. Remove it from the stove, and put the pan in the oven. Let it cook for forty-five minutes.
7. Allow it to sit for ten minutes before serving.

Green Beans with Sesame Pork

Serves: 2

Time: 15 Minutes

Calories: 366

Protein: 33 Grams

Fiber: 2 Grams

Fat: 24 Grams

Net Carbs: 3 Grams

Ingredients:

- 1 Cup Green Beans, Fresh
- 2 Pork Chops, Boneless
- 2 Tablespoons Toasted Sesame Oil, Divided
- 2 Tablespoons Soy Sauce
- 1 Teaspoon Sriracha Sauce

Directions:

1. Pat your pork dry using a paper towel before slicing it into strips. Season as desired.
2. Place a large skillet over medium heat, adding in a tablespoon of your sesame oil.
3. Add the pork to your skillet, allowing it to cook for seven minutes. You will need to stir occasionally.
4. Take out a small bowl, whisking together your Sriracha sauce, soy sauce and sesame oil before pouring the mixture over your sliced pork.
5. Add your green beans in, reducing the heat to medium-low. Allow everything to simmer for three to five minutes.
6. Serve warm.

Crockpot BBQ Ribs

Serves: 2

Time: 4 Hours 10 Minutes

Calories: 956

Protein: 68 Grams

Fiber: 0 Grams

Fat: 72 Grams

Net Carbs: 5 Grams

Ingredients:

- 1 lb. Pork Ribs
- 1.25 Ounces Dry Rib Seasoning Rub
- ½ Cup Barbecue Sauce, Sugar Free
- Sea Salt & Black Pepper to Taste

Directions:

1. Start by turning your crockpot to high, and then season your pork ribs with your dry rib seasoning rub, salt and pepper.
2. Stand them up in your crockpot with the bone side facing inward, and then pour the barbecue sauce over them. Make sure that you coat both sides, but don't put too much into your crockpot.
3. Allow it to cook while covered for four hours before serving warm.

Blue Cheese Pork Chops

Serves: 2

Time: 15 Minutes

Calories: 669

Protein: 41 Grams

Fiber: 0 Grams

Fat: 34 Grams

Net Carbs: 4 Grams

Ingredients:

- 2 Tablespoons Butter
- 2 Pork Chops, Boneless
- 1/3 Cup Heavy Whipping Cream
- 1/3 Cup Blue Cheese, Crumbled
- 1/3 Cup Sour Cream

Directions:

1. Start by patting your pork chops dry and seasoning them if desired.
2. Place a skillet over medium heat, and then melt the butter. Once your butter is hot, then add in the pork chops, cooking or three minutes on each side.
3. Take a saucepan, placing it over medium heat and then melt your blue cheese. Make sure that you stir frequently, and then add in your cream and sour cream. Allow the mixture to simmer or a few minutes while you continue to stir.
4. Add in the juice from the pork chops, pouring it into your pan and stir well. Allow it to simmer.
5. Plate your pork chops and pour the blue cheese sauce over it.

Chapter 5: Side Dishes Recipes

Spicy Butter Beans

Serves: 4

Time: 15 Minutes

Calories: 93

Protein: 2 Grams

Fiber: 4 Grams

Fat: 8 Grams

Net Carbs: 4 Grams

Ingredients:

- 2 Cloves Garlic, Minced
- Red Pepper Flakes to Taste
- Sea Salt to Taste
- 2 Tablespoons Golden Ghee
- 4 Cups Green Beans, Trimmed

Directions:

1. Bring a pot of water to a boil, adding sea salt. Once the water starts to boil, cook your green beans for three minutes.
2. Prepare a bowl of ice water, and then drain your green beans and plunge them into the ice water. This will stop them from cooking, and then once they're cooled, drain them again, placing them to the side.
3. Take a medium skillet, and then melt your ghee using medium heat. Once your ghee is hot, add your red pepper, sea salt and garlic. Cook until your garlic is soft and fragrant. This should take about a minute.
4. Add in your green beans, tossing until they're coated. This should take another three minutes.

5. Serve warm.

Blue Cheese Zoodles with Bacon

Serves: 1

Time: 10 Minutes

Calories: 435

Protein: 21 Grams

Fiber: 1 Gram

Fat: 33 Grams

Net Carbs: 5 Grams

Ingredients:

- ½ Cup Baby Spinach, Fresh
- 1 Cup Zucchini, Spiralized & Cold
- ½ Cup Bacon, Cooked & Crumbled
- 1/3 Cup Blue Cheese, Crumbled
- 3 Tablespoons Blue Cheese Dressing, Chunky

Directions:

1. Toss everything together in a large bowl before serving cool.

Buttery Mushrooms

Serves: 2

Time: 4 Hours 10 Minutes

Calories: 351

Protein: 6 Grams

Fiber: 1 Gram

Fat: 36 Grams

Net Carbs: 4 Grams

Ingredients:

- 6 Tablespoons Butter
- 8 Ounces cremini Mushrooms, Fresh
- 1 Tablespoon Italian Parsley, Fresh & Chopped
- 2 Tablespoons Parmesan Cheese, Grated
- 1 Tablespoon Ranch Dressing Mix

Directions:

1. Start by preheating your slow cooker, and ten mix your butter and dry ranch together at the bottom. Allow your butter to completely melt.
2. Add in your mushrooms, making sure they're coated. Sprinkle them with your parmesan.
3. Put the lid on, and allow it to cook on low for four hours.
4. Use a slotted spoon to serve. Sprinkle your chopped parsley on top before serving.

Asparagus & Walnuts

Serves: 4

Time: 15 Minutes

Calories: 124

Protein: 3 Grams

Fiber: 2 Grams

Fat: 12 Grams

Net Carbs: 2 Grams

Ingredients:

- 1 ½ Tablespoons Olive Oil
- ¾ lb. Asparagus, Trimmed
- ¼ Cup Walnuts, Chopped
- Sea Salt & Black Pepper to Taste

Directions:

1. Put a skillet over medium-high heat, adding in your olive oil.
2. Add in your asparagus, sautéing until they're tender and browned slightly. This should take about five minutes.
3. Season it with your salt and pepper, and then remove it from the skillet.
4. Toss your walnuts with the asparagus, and serve warm.

Cheesy Brussel Sprouts

Serves: 8

Time: 45 Minutes

Calories: 299

Protein: 12 Grams

Fiber: 3 Grams

Fat: 11 Grams

Net Carbs: 4 Grams

Ingredients:

- 8 Slices Bacon
- 1 lb. Brussel Sprouts, Blanched & Quartered
- 1 Cup Swiss Cheese, Shredded & Divided
- ¾ Cup Heavy Whipping Cream

Directions:

1. Start by heating your oven to 400.
2. Put your skillet over medium-high heat, adding in your bacon. Cook for six minutes or until it's crispy.
3. Reserve a tablespoon of your grease, greasing your casserole dish with it. Chop your cooked bacon.
4. Take out a bowl and toss your chopped bacon with your Brussel sprouts.
5. Add in a half a cup of your cheese, and mix well before transferring it to your casserole dish.
6. Pour your cream over it, and top it with the remaining cheese.
7. Bake your casserole for twenty minutes, and serve warm.

Creamed Spinach

Serves: 3

Time: 15 Minutes

Calories: 248

Protein: 10.9 Grams

Fiber: 4.4 Grams

Fat: 20.5 Grams

Net Carbs: 3.7 Grams

Ingredients:

- 1.3 lbs. Spinach, fresh
- 1/3 Cup Mascarpone Cheese
- ¼ Teaspoon Nutmeg
- 2 Tablespoon Butter
- 1/3 Cup Parmesan Cheese, Grated
- Sea Salt (Optional)

Directions:

1. Start by bringing a pot of water to boil, using it to blanch your spinach for thirty to sixty seconds. Then plunge your spinach in ice water, draining it and setting it to the side.
2. Put your mascarpone and butter in a pan, adding in your spinach. Season if desired with salt, and then add in your nutmeg. Gently bring it to a simmer.
3. Mix your parmesan in before serving.

Camembert Mushrooms

Serves: 4

Time: 20 Minutes

Calories: 161

Protein: 9 Grams

Fiber: 1 Gram

Fat: 13 Grams

Net Carbs: 3 Grams

Ingredients:

- 2 Tablespoons Butter
- 4 Ounces Camembert Cheese, Diced
- 2 Teaspoons Garlic, Minced
- 1 lb. Button Mushrooms, Halved
- Black Pepper to Taste

Directions:

1. Put a skillet over medium-high heat, adding in your butter. Once your butter has melted, add in your garlic. Sauté it until it becomes translucent, which should take about three minutes.
2. Add in your mushrooms, cooking until they're tender. It should take about ten minutes, and then season with pepper before serving.

Bacon & Broccoli Salad

Serves: 2

Time: 1 Hour 20 Minutes

Calories: 549

Protein: 16 Grams

Fiber: 5 Grams

Fat: 49 Grams

Net Carbs: 11 Grams

Ingredients:

- 6 Slices Bacon
- ½ lb. Broccoli, Fresh & Chopped into Florets
- ¼ Cup Almonds, Sliced
- 1/3 Cup Mayonnaise
- 1 Tablespoon Honey Mustard Dressing

Directions:

1. Place a skillet over medium-high heat. Cook your bacon until its brown and crisp, which should take about eight minutes.
2. Place your bacon a paper towel so that I drains for about five minutes, and then crumble it.
3. In a bowl combine your bacon, almonds and broccoli.
4. Mix your mayonnaise and honey mustard together, adding in your dressing. Toss to combine.
5. Chill for an hour.

Roasted Broccoli

Serves: 4

Time: 40 Minutes

Calories: 62.25

Protein: 4.35 Grams

Fiber: 2.53 Grams

Fat: 3.73 Grams

Net Carbs: 3.89 Grams

Ingredients:

- 4 Cups Broccoli Florets
- 1 Tablespoon Olive Oil
- Sea Salt & Black Pepper to Taste

Directions:

1. Start by heating your oven to 400, putting your broccoli in a zipper top bag with your oil. Shake until coated well.
2. Add in your seasoning, shaking again.
3. Spread the broccoli out on the baking sheet, baking for twenty to thirty minutes. It should be crisp.
4. Allow it to cool before serving.

Parmesan Green Beans

Serves: 3

Time: 35 Minutes

Calories: 221.05

Protein: 3.44 Grams

Fiber: 4.2 Grams

Fat: 9.16 Grams

Net Carbs: 7.47 Grams

Ingredients:

- 1 lb. Green Beans, Fresh & Stems Removed
- 1 Tablespoon Olive Oil
- 1 Tablespoon Butter, Unsalted
- 2 Cloves Garlic, Minced
- 1 Tablespoon Parmesan Cheese
- Sea Salt (Optional)

Directions:

1. Fill a bowl with water and ice, setting it to the side as you bring a pot of water to boil on the stove.
2. Add your green beans to the water once it starts to boil, steaming them for about four minutes.
3. Drain them immediately before plunging them in the ice water to stop the cooking.
4. Allow your green beans to cool, and place a pan over medium heat. Melt your butter, and then add in your garlic and olive oil.
5. Drain your green beans, and then add them into the pan once your garlic begins to sizzle. Make sure that they're coated in the oil.
6. Season if desired, and then remove them from heat.
7. Sprinkle with parmesan cheese before serving.

Keto Mash

Serves: 4

Time: 15 Minutes

Calories: 302

Protein: 3.7 Grams

Fiber: 3.8 Grams

Fat: 28 Grams

Net Carbs: 7 Grams

Ingredients:

- 1 Cauliflower, Large
- 2 Cloves Garlic, Minced
- 1 White Onion, Small
- ½ Cup Ghee
- Sea Salt to Taste

Directions:

1. Start by washing your cauliflower before chopping it into florets.
2. Bring a pot of water to a boil, cooking your florets for ten minutes. Make sure that you don't overcook them.
3. Grease a pan with two tablespoons of the ghee, adding in your garlic and onion over medium heat. Cook until slightly brown, which should take about five minutes. You'll need to keep stirring to keep it from burning.
4. Remove the mixture from heat, and then add your cauliflower into a blender, blending until creamy and smooth.
5. Add in your garlic mixture, blending again.
6. Stir well, and then serve topped with butter.

Turnip Fries

Serves: 4

Time: 35 Minutes

Calories: 129

Protein: 1.7 Grams

Fiber: 3.3 Grams

Fat: 9.5 Grams

Net Carbs: 7.7 Grams

Ingredients:

- 2 lbs. Turnips
- ¼ Cup Olive Oil
- 2 Tablespoons Taco Seasoning
- 2 Teaspoons Sea Salt, Fine

Directions:

1. Start by heating your oven to 350, and then wash your turnips before patting them dry. Peel them, discarding the peel.
2. Slice your turnips into half inch sticks.
3. Put your turnip slices in a zipper top bag, adding in your sea salt, taco seasoning and oil, zipping it up and tossing to coat.
4. Line a baking sheet with parchment paper, placing your turnip sticks in a single layer.
5. Bake until golden brown, but make sure that you do not overbake them. This usually takes about twenty-five minutes.

Pink Sauerkraut

Serves: 14

Time: 1 Week 15 Minutes

Calories: 8

Protein: 0.4 Grams

Fiber: 1 Gram

Fat: 0.1 Grams

Net Carbs: 0.8 Grams

Ingredients:

- 1 lb. Cabbage, Grated
- 1 Beetroot, Small
- 1 Teaspoon Ginger, Fresh & Grated
- 1 Teaspoon Sea Salt, Fine

Directions:

1. Core and finely slice your red cabbage, and then peel and grate your beetroot.
2. Grate your ginger, and then add it to the mixture. Sprinkle it with salt, and then place the mixture in a glass jar. Pound it down so that it is using a spoon. It should release juices as you pack it down. It should have enough juices to cover your mixture. If there isn't, then set it aside for eight hours before pressing it again.
3. Cover the jar with a cloth and secure it somewhere where there is a stable temperature. Allow it to sit for a week, and then place it in the fridge to slow the fermentation down.

Braised Fennel with Lemon

Serves: 6

Time: 1 Hour 45 Minutes

Calories: 128

Protein: 1.9 Grams

Fiber: 4.7 Grams

Fat: 9.3 Grams

Net Carbs: 6.8

Ingredients:

- 2 lbs. Fennel Bulbs
- ¼ Cup Olive Oil
- 3 Lemons, Large
- Sea Salt to Taste

Directions:

1. Start by heating your oven to 375, and then cut your fennel bulbs into wedges.
2. Slice your lemons thin, and then arrange your fennel and lemons in a fifteen by ten inch baking dish.
3. Drizzle your oil over it before covering it with foil.
4. Cook for an hour, and then uncover before cooking or another twenty-five to forty minutes. It should be golden and crisp, and then remove to cool.

Bacon Snap Peas

Serves: 4

Time: 15 Minutes

Calories: 147.33

Protein: 1.95 Grams

Fiber: 1.77 Grams

Fat: 13.04 Grams

Net Carbs: 4.33 Grams

Ingredients:

- 3 Tablespoons Bacon Fat
- 2 Teaspoons Garlic, Minced
- ½ Teaspoon Red Pepper Flakes
- ½ Lemon, Large & Juiced
- 3 Cups Sugar Snap Peas

Directions:

1. Start by adding your bacon fat to a pan, bringing it up to your smoking point
2. Add the garlic, reducing the heat. Allow it to cook for one to two minutes before adding in your sugar snap peas. Season with lemon juice, cooking for another two minutes.
3. Serve garnished with your lemon zest and red pepper flakes.

Bacon Jam Green Beans

Serves: 3

Time: 15 Minutes

Calories: 158.55

Protein: 4.81 Grams

Fiber: 3.95 Grams

Fat: 11.31 Grams

Net Carbs: 6.88 Grams

Ingredients:

- 1 Tablespoon Olive Oil
- 2 ½ Cups Green Beans, Fresh
- 3 Tablespoons Bacon Jam

Directions:

1. Start by brining your water to a boil, adding your green beans in. blanch them for three to four minutes.
2. Drain them, and then place them in an ice bath for about three minutes
3. In a pan take your jam and olive oil, heating it up.
4. Drain your green beans again, and then dry them before adding them to the pan.
5. Stir everything together, cooking for another two minutes.
6. Serve warm.

Cauliflower & Cheese Casserole

Serves: 8

Time: 40 Minutes

Calories: 135.13

Protein: 5.42 Grams

Fiber: 1.59 Grams

Fat: 10.48 Grams

Net Carbs: 4.47 Grams

Ingredients:

- 1 Cup Sour Cream
- 1 Cup Cheddar Cheese, Shredded
- ½ Onion, Chopped
- 1 Head Cauliflower
- Sea Salt to Taste

Directions:

1. Chop your cauliflower, putting it in the casserole dish.
2. Dice your onions, tossing it in with your cauliflowers.
3. Pour the cheese and sour cream in before mixing.
4. Heat your oven to 350, and bake it for a half hour.
5. Serve warm.

Zucchini Gratin

Serves: 2

Time: 1 Hour

Calories: 355

Protein: 28 Grams

Fiber: 2 Grams

Fat: 25 Grams

Net Carbs: 4 Grams

Ingredients:

- 1 Zucchini, Sliced Thin
- 1 Ounce Brie Cheese, Rind Trimmed
- 1 Tablespoon Butter
- ¼ Cup Pork Rinds
- 1/3 Cup Gruyere Cheese, Shredded (optional)
- Sea Salt

Directions:

1. Stat by slicing your zucchini and salting it so that the excess water gets pulled out.
2. Preheat your oven to 400, and then put a pan over medium-low heat. Place your butter and Brie in it, and then cook until it's melted.
3. Place your zucchini in a baking dish so that the slices are overlapping, seasoning it as desired.
4. Pour your brie mixture over your zucchini, and then top with Gruyere cheese if desired.
5. Crush your pork rinds, sprinkling it on top.
6. Allow the dish to bake for twenty-five minutes. It should be browned on top and bubbly.

Brussel Sprouts & Bacon

Serves: 2

Time: 30 Minutes

Calories: 248

Protein: 14 Grams

Fiber: 5 Grams

Fat: 18 Grams

Net Carbs: 7 Grams

Ingredients:

- ½ lb. Brussel Sprouts, Trimmed & Halved
- 1 Tablespoon Olive Oil
- 1 Teaspoon Red Pepper Flakes
- 6 Bacon Slices
- 1 Tablespoon Parmesan Cheese
- Sea Salt (Optional)

Directions:

1. Start by heating your oven to 400 and take out a small bowl.
2. Combine your Brussel sprouts and olive oil together. Season with red pepper flakes and salt if desired.
3. Chop your bacon into one inch pieces, and then spread your Brussel sprouts and bacon on a baking sheet. Make sure it's a single layer.
4. Cook for twenty-five minutes, making sure to stir halfway through. They should be crisp and brown.
5. Sprinkle with parmesan cheese before serving.

Prosciutto Brussel Sprouts & Leeks

Serves: 6

Time: 30 Minutes

Calories: 177.25

Protein: 5.66 Grams

Fiber: 1.88 Grams

Fat: 15.16 Grams

Net Carbs: 3.64 Grams

Ingredients:

- ½ Cup Leeks
- ¼ Cup Coconut Oil
- 1 Cup Prosciutto, Chopped
- 2 Cups Brussels Sprouts

Directions:

1. Wash your leeks, slicing them thin. Rinse them, and then drain them.
2. Trim your Brussel sprouts before halving them.
3. Place a skillet over medium heat, adding in your coconut oil, and then add in your leeks and Brussel sprouts. Allow them to brown.
4. Add in your prosciutto, and then cover the lid. Reduce the heat to low, cooking for ten more minutes.
5. Mix well before serving.

Pork Rind & Parmesan Green Beans

Serves: 2

Time: 20 Minutes

Calories: 175

Protein: 6 Grams

Fiber: 3 Grams

Fat: 15 Grams

Net Carbs: 5 Grams

Ingredients:

- 2 Tablespoons Olive Oil
- ½ lb. Green Beans, Fresh
- 2 Tablespoons Pork Rinds, Crushed
- 1 Tablespoon Parmesan Cheese, Grated
- Sea Salt to Taste

Directions:

1. Start by heating your oven to 400.
2. Combine your pork rinds, olive oil, green beans and parmesan cheese together. Season with salt, and then toss your green beans to make sure that they're coated thoroughly.
3. Spread the mixture on a baking sheet in a single layer, roasting for fifteen minutes. Halfway through, make sure to stir your green beans.
4. Allow it to cool before serving.

Roasted Radishes in a Butter Sauce

Serves: 2

Time: 25 Minutes

Calories: 181

Protein: 1 Gram

Fiber: 2 Grams

Fat: 19 Grams

Net Carbs: 2 Grams

Ingredients:

- 1 Tablespoon Olive Oil
- Sea Salt to Taste
- 2 Tablespoons Butter
- 1 Tablespoon Parsley, fresh & Chopped
- 2 Cups Radishes, Halved

Directions:

1. Start by heating your oven to 450, and then take out a bowl. Toss your radishes in your olive oil, seasoning with salt.
2. Lay your radishes in a baking sheet in a single layer, and then roast it for fifteen minutes. Make sure to stir eight minutes in.
3. In a saucepan over medium heat, melt your butter, seasoning with more salt. As it begins to bubble and foam, you need to continue stirring. Your butter should turn a light brown, and then you place it to the side.
4. Take your radishes from the oven, and then serve with your browned butter.

Chapter 6: Dessert Recipes

Coffee Popsicles

Serves: 4

Time: 2 Hours 5 Minutes

Calories: 105

Portion: 1 Gram

Fiber: 2 Grams

Fat: 10 Grams

Net Carbs: 2 Grams

Ingredients:

- 2 Tablespoons Chocolate Chips, Sugar Free
- 2 Cups Coffee, Brewed & Cold
- ¾ Cup Heavy Whipping Cream
- 2 Teaspoons Natural Sweetener

Directions:

1. Blend your heavy whipping cream, sweetener and coffee in a blender.
2. Pour the mixture into your Popsicle mold, and then add a few chocolate chips into each.
3. Allow it to freeze for at least two hours before serving.

Easy Chocolate Mousse

Serves: 2

Time: 1 Hour 10 Minutes

Calories: 460

Protein: 4 Grams

Fiber: 1 Gram

Fat: 50 Grams

Net Carbs: 4 Grams

Ingredients:

- 1 Tablespoon Natural Sweetener
- 1 ½ Tablespoons Heavy Whipping Cream
- 1 Tablespoon Cocoa Powder, Unsweetened
- 4 Tablespoons Butter, Room Temperature
- 4 Tablespoons Cream Cheese, Room Temperature

Directions:

1. Chill a bowl, and whisk your cream in it until it's whipped. Put it in the fridge to keep it cold.
2. In another bowl, mix your cocoa powder, sweetener, butter and cream cheese together with a hand mixer.
3. Take the whipped cream out, folding it into the chocolate mixture. Make sure to scrape the sides as needed, and then divide it between bowls.
4. Cover the bowls, and then chill it for at least an hour before serving.

Berry Ice Popsicles

Serves: 2

Time: 2 Hours 5 Minutes

Calories: 165

Protein: 1 Gram

Fiber: 1 Gram

Fat: 17 Grams

Net Carbs: 2 Grams

Ingredients:

- ½ Can Coconut Cream, Canned
- 2 Teaspoons Natural Sweetener
- ½ Teaspoon Vanilla Extract
- ¼ Cup Mixed Blackberries & Blueberries

Directions:

1. Take a blender, mixing your sweetener, vanilla and coconut cream together.
2. Add in your berries, pulsing until mostly smooth.
3. Pour this mixture into your Popsicle mold, allowing it to freeze before serving.

Keto Root Beer Float

Serves: 2

Time: 5 Minutes

Calories: 56

Protein: 1 Gram

Fiber: 0 Grams

Fat: 6 Grams

Net Carbs: 1 Gram

Ingredients:

- 6 Ice Cubes
- 12 Ounces Root Beer, Diet
- 4 Tablespoons Heavy Whipping Cream
- 1 Teaspoon Vanilla Extract

Directions:

1. Blend your cream, vanilla, ice and root beer together, and then pour it in a glass to serve.

Easy Strawberry Shake

Serves: 2

Time: 10 Minutes

Calories: 407

Protein: 4 Grams

Fiber: 1 Gram

Fat: 42 Grams

Net Carbs: 6 Grams

Ingredients:

- 6 Strawberries, Sliced
- 6 Ice Cubes
- ¼ Teaspoon Vanilla Extract (Optional)
- 1 Tablespoon Natural Sweetener
- 2 Ounces Cream Cheese, Room Temperature
- ¾ Cup Heavy Whipping Cream

Directions:

1. Blend all ingredients together until smooth, and serve immediately.

Chocolate & Mint Ice Cream

Serves: 2

Time: 4 Hours 40 Minutes

Calories: 325

Protein: 3 Grams

Fiber: 4 Grams

Fat: 33 Grams

Net Carbs: 4 Grams

Ingredients:

- 2 Tablespoons Chocolate Chips, Sugar Free
- ¼ Teaspoon Peppermint Extract
- ½ Tablespoon Butter
- 1 Tablespoon Natural Sweetener
- 10 Tablespoons Heavy Whipping Cream, Divided

Directions:

1. Take out a saucepan, putting it over medium heat. Melt the butter, whisking in your sweetener and five tablespoons of your cream.
2. Turn the heat up to medium-high, bringing it to a boil. Stir it constantly while you do this, and then turn it down to low. Allow it to simmer while you stir occasionally for a half hour. The mixture should be stick so that it sticks to the back of the spoon.
3. Add in your peppermint extract, mixing well.
4. Pour your thickened mixture into a bowl, and refrigerate it to cool it down.
5. Remove your metal bowl, and it may be best to put your mixer beaters in the freezer for this part. Pour your remaining cream into your bowl, and whip it until it's fluffy and forms peaks. Make sure you don't overbeat it or your cream will turn into butter. Take your cream mix out of the fridge.

6. Gently fold your whipped cream into your cooled mix, and then transfer it to a metal container.
7. Mix your chocolate chips in, and then cover the container.
8. Freeze your ice cream for four to five hours before serving. You'll need to stir it twice during this time.

Easy Peanut Butter Cookies

Serves: 15

Time: 25 Minutes

Calories: 98

Protein: 4 Grams

Fiber: 1 Gram

Fat: 8 Grams

Net Carbs: 3 Grams

Ingredients:

- 1 Egg
- ½ Cup Natural Sweetener
- 1 Cup Peanut Butter, Natural & Crunchy

Directions:

1. Start by heating your oven to 350, and then take out a baking sheet. Line it with parchment paper.
2. Take out a bowl and mix your peanut butter, egg and sweetener together.
3. Roll it into balls that are about an inch in diameter.
4. Spread it on your cookie sheet, flattening the balls with a fork to create a crisscross pattern.
5. Bake it for twelve minutes. Your cookies should be golden, and you will want to let them cool for ten minutes before serving. They'll store in the fridge for up to five days.

Lime & Strawberry Popsicles

Serves: 4

Time: 2 Hours 5 Minutes

Calories: 166

Protein: 1 Gram

Fiber: 1 Gram

Fat: 17 Grams

Net Carbs: 3 Grams

Ingredients:

- 1 Tablespoon Lime Juice, Fresh
- ¼ Cup Strawberries, Hulled & Sliced
- ¾ Cup Coconut Milk, Unsweetened & Full Fat
- 2 Teaspoons Natural Sweetener

Directions:

1. Add your coconut milk, sweetener, and lime juice in a blender. Blend until smooth, and then add in your strawberries pulse until mostly smooth.
2. Pour the mixture into your Popsicle mold, and then freeze for at least two hours before serving.

Avocado & Chocolate Pudding

Serves: 2

Time: 35 Minutes

Calories: 281

Protein: 8 Grams

Fiber: 10 Grams

Fat: 27 Grams

Net Carbs: 12 Grams

Ingredients:

- 1 Avocado, Chunked
- 1 Tablespoon Natural Sweetener
- 2 Ounces Cream Cheese, Room Temperature
- ¼ Teaspoon Vanilla Extract
- 4 Tablespoons Cocoa Powder, Unsweetened

Directions:

1. Blend all of your ingredients until smooth in a blender.
2. Divide the mixture between dessert bowls, chilling for a half hour before serving.

Lemonade Fat Bomb

Serves: 2

Time: 2 Hours 10 Minutes

Calories: 404

Protein: 4 Grams

Fiber: 1 Gram

Fat: 43 Grams

Net Carbs: 4 Grams

Ingredients:

- ½ Lemon
- 4 Ounces Cream Cheese, Room Temperature
- 2 Ounces Butter, Room Temperature
- Pink Sea Salt to Taste
- 2 Teaspoons Natural Sweetener

Directions:

1. Take a fine grater and zest your lemon, squeezing the juice into the bowl with your zest.
2. Combine your butter and cream cheese in a butter, adding in your lemon zest, juice, pink sea salt, and your sweetener. Use a hand mixer to combine the mixture until smooth.
3. Spoon this mixture into molds, and then allow it to freeze for two hours.

Fudge Popsicles

Serves: 4

Time: 2 Hours 5 Minutes

Calories: 193

Protein: 2 Grams

Fiber: 3 Grams

Fat: 20 Grams

Net Carbs: 3 Grams

Ingredients:

- 2 Tablespoons Cocoa Powder, Unsweetened
- 2 Tablespoons Chocolate Chips, Sugar Free
- 2 Teaspoons Natural Sweetener
- ¾ Cup Heavy Whipping Cream

Directions:

1. Blend your coconut cream, unsweetened cocoa powder and sweetener together until smooth.
2. Pour it into your Popsicle molds, and then drop some chocolate chips into it.
3. Allow it to freeze for at least two hours before serving.

Easy Strawberry Bark

Serves: 2

Time: 2 Hours 15 Minutes

Calories: 111

Protein: 3 Grams

Fiber: 5 Grams

Fat: 10 Grams

Net Carbs: 4 Grams

Ingredients:

- 1 Strawberry, Fresh & Sliced
- 1 Tablespoon Heavy Whipping Cream
- 2 Tablespoons Almonds, Salted
- ½ Chocolate Bar, Keto Friendly

Directions:

1. Take out a baking sheet, lining it with parchment paper.
2. Break the chocolate into small pieces, and then heat it in a microwave safe bowl with cream, mixing well. Heat it for forty-five seconds the first time and then twenty second intervals until mixed well.
3. Pour the mixture over your parchment paper to form a thin layer.
4. Sprinkle your almonds and strawberries on top, and then refrigerate it for about two hours until hardened.
5. Break it up into smaller pieces, and serve chilled.
6. It can keep for four days in the fridge.

Toffee Nut Cups

Serves: 5

Time: 1 Hour 15 Minutes

Calories: 194.4

Protein: 2.5 Grams

Fiber: 6.18 Grams

Fat: 18.76 Grams

Net Carbs: 2.21 Grams

Ingredients:

- 5 Ounces Milk Chocolate, Low Carb
- ½ Ounce Walnuts, Raw & Chopped
- Sea Salt to Taste
- 3 Tablespoons Butter, Cold
- 3 Tablespoons + @ Teaspoons Erythritol

Directions:

1. Microwave your chocolate in forty-five second intervals, stirring frequently until it's melted.
2. Put five cupcake liners in a muffin tin, dropping some chocolate into each. Makes sure it evenly covers the bottom, and then brush it up the edges using a pastry brush. Freeze it until it hardens.
3. Take out a microwave safe glass bowl, heating your cold butter and Erythritol for three minutes, and then mix it every twenty seconds to keep it from burning. It's okay for it to look watery, and then add two teaspoons of your Erythritol, stirring it until it thickens. Add in your walnuts, and then remove the cups from the freezer. Reheat the chocolate if you need to, and fill each cup with a half a spoon of your toffee mix.
4. Top your cups with chocolate chips, placing the cups in the fridge for an hour.
5. Sprinkle with sea salt before serving.

Very Berry Cheesecake Fat Bombs

Serves: 2

Time: 2 Hours 10 Minutes

Calories: 414

Protein: 4 Grams

Fiber: 1 Gram

Fat: 43 Grams

Net Carbs: 4 Grams

Ingredients:

- 2 Teaspoons natural Sweetener
- 1 Teaspoon Vanilla Extract
- ¼ Cup Berries, Fresh
- 4 Tablespoons Butter, Room Temperature
- 4 Ounces Cream Cheese, Room Temperature

Directions:

1. Take a bowl and mix your butter, vanilla, sweetener and cream cheese, mixing it well.
2. In a bowl mix mash your berries, and then old it into your cream cheese mixture.
3. Spoon this mixture into fat bomb molds, and then freeze or a minimum of two hours before serving.

Pecan & Berry Mascarpone Bowl

Serves: 2

Time: 5 Minutes

Calories: 462

Protein: 6 Grams

Fiber: 7 Grams

Fat: 47 Grams

Net Carbs: 6 Grams

Ingredients:

- 1 Teaspoon Natural Sweetener
- ¼ Cup Mascarpone
- 6 Strawberries, Fresh & Sliced
- 30 Dark Chocolate Chips
- 1 Cup Pecans, Chopped

Directions:

1. Divide the pecans between two bowls, and then take out another bowl for mixing.
2. Mix your sweetener and mascarpone cheese, making sure it's well combined. Top your pecans with a dollop of the mascarpone, and then sprinkle your chocolate chips over each bowl.
3. Divide your strawberries between the bowls, and then serve.

Creamy Orange Soda Float

Serves: 2

Time: 5 Minutes

Calories: 56

Protein: 1 Gram

Fiber: 0 Grams

Fat: 6 Grams

Net Carbs: 1 Gram

Ingredients:

- 6 Ice Cubes
- 1 Can Orange Soda, Diet
- 4 Tablespoons Heavy Whipping Cream
- 1 Teaspoon Vanilla Extract

Directions:

1. Blend all ingredients in a food processor until smooth, and then serve immediately.

Easy Chocolate Shake

Serves: 2

Time: 1 Hour 10 Minutes

Calories: 444

Protein: 4 Grams

Fiber: 2 Grams

Fat: 47 Grams

Net Carbs: 7 Grams

Ingredients:

- ¼ Teaspoon Vanilla Extract
- 2 Tablespoons Cocoa Powder, Unsweetened
- ¾ Cup Heavy Whipping Cream
- 4 Ounces Coconut Milk
- 1 Tablespoon Natural Sweetener

Directions:

1. Chill a metal bowl, and pour your cream in it. Add your vanilla, cocoa powder, and sweetener. Blend until it's fully combined, and then pour in your coconut milk. Gently stir, and then add your cocoa powder, sweetener and vanilla together until it's fully combined.
2. Pour it into two glasses, and then let it freeze for an hour before serving.

Meringue Cookies

Serves: 18

Time: 1 Hour 5 Minutes

Calories: 4.11

Protein: 0.8 Grams

Fiber: 0 Grams

Fat: 0.01 Grams

Net Carbs: 0.09 Grams

Ingredients:

- 4 Egg Whites, Large
- 6 Tablespoons Swerve Confectioners
- ½ Teaspoon Almond Extract
- ¼ Teaspoon Cream of Tartar
- Pinch Sea Salt, Fine

Directions:

1. Start by heating your oven to 210, pouring your egg whites into a mixing bowl. Add in your cream of tartar, mixing slow on medium speed, and the egg whites should become frothy. Add in three tablespoons of your swerve, your sea salt and your almond extract
2. Mix it on high speed until the egg whites whip up. They should have a medium consistency, and then add the remaining Swerve.
3. Continue to whip on high until it becomes stiff. It should start to pull away from the sides, and make sure everything is mixed evenly.
4. Put it in a piping bag, fitting it with a star shaped tip. You'll want to use a large tip, and you may need to fill your bag more than once
5. Take out two to three baking sheets, lining them with parchment paper. Pope out eight shapes, and then bake them for forty minutes. Turn the oven of, and then crack the oven door open. Let them cool for a half hour before serving.

Crust Free Pumpkin Cheesecake Bites

Serves: 4

Time: 3 Hours 40 Minutes

Calories: 156

Protein: 5 Grams

Fiber: 1 Gram

Fat: 12 Grams

Net Carbs: 4 Grams

Ingredients:

- 4 Ounces Pumpkin Puree
- 2 Eggs, Large
- 2 Teaspoons Pumpkin Pie Spice
- 1/3 Cup Natural Sweetener
- 4 Ounces Cream Cheese, Room Temperature

Directions:

1. Start by turning your oven to 350, and then take out a bowl.
2. Mix your pumpkin puree, cream cheese, eggs, pumpkin pie spice and sweetener until completely mixed
3. Put some paper cupcake liners in a muffin tin, pouring in your batter.
4. Bake it for a half hour, and then refrigerate it for at least three hours before serving. These will keep for up to three months in the freezer.

Peanut Butter Fat Bomb

Serves: 2

Time: 40 Minutes

Calories: 196

Protein: 3 Grams

Fiber: 1 Gram

Fat: 20 Grams

Net Carbs: 3 Grams

Ingredients:

- 2 Teaspoons Natural Sweetener
- 1 Tablespoon Butter, Room Temperature
- 1 Tablespoons Coconut Oil
- 2 Tablespoons Peanut Butter, All Natural

Directions:

1. Melt your coconut oil, peanut butter and butter in a microwave safe bowl, and mix in your sweetener. Make sure it's well combined, and then pour the mixture into fat bomb molds.
2. Allow it to freeze for a half an hour before serving.

Strawberry Cheesecake Mousse

Serves: 2

Time: 1 Hour 10 Minutes

Calories: 221

Protein: 4 Grams

Fiber: 1 Gram

Fat: 21 Grams

Net Carbs: 4 Grams

Ingredients:

- 1 Teaspoon Vanilla Extract
- 4 Strawberries, Fresh & Sliced
- 4 Ounces Cream Cheese, Room Temperature
- 1 Tablespoon Heavy Whipping Cream
- 1 Teaspoon Natural Sweetener

Directions:

1. Break up the cream cheese, and then place it in your blender. Add in your sweetener, vanilla and cream. Blend on high, and make sure that you scrape the sides. Continue to blend until smooth.
2. Add in your strawberries, blending again.
3. Divide the mixture between two dishes, chilling for about an hour before serving.

Peanut Butter & Coconut Balls

Serves: 15

Time: 1 Hour 10 Minutes

Calories: 35.13

Protein: 0.98 Grams

Fiber: 0.59 Grams

Fat: 3.19 Grams

Net Carbs: 0.92 Grams

Ingredients:

- ½ Cup Coconut Flakes, Unsweetened
- 2 Teaspoons Almond Flour
- 2 ½ Teaspoons Powdered Erythritol
- 3 Tablespoons Creamy Peanut Butter
- 3 Teaspoons Cocoa Powder, Unsweetened

Directions:

1. Take out a bowl and mix your cocoa powder, Erythritol, flour and peanut butter together.
2. Freeze it for an hour, and then use a melon baller to make scoops. Drop it in your coconut flakes, rolling it until they're covered.
3. Keep it in the fridge overnight, and serve cold.

Crust Free Cheesecake Bites

Serves: 4

Time: 3 Hours 40 Minutes

Calories: 169

Protein: 5 Grams

Fiber: 0 Grams

Fat: 15 Grams

Net Carbs: 2 Grams

Ingredients:

- ¼ Teaspoon Vanilla Extract
- 2 Eggs, Large
- 4 Ounces Cream Cheese, Room Temperature
- 1/3 Cup Natural Sweetener
- ¼ Cup Sour Cream

Directions:

1. Start by heating your oven to 350, and then take out a bowl.
2. Beat your eggs, sweetener, sour cream, vanilla and cream cheese until combined.
3. Take out a muffin tin, lining it with paper liners, and then pour the batter into the liners.
4. Bake it for a half an hour, and then place it in the fridge or three hours. They'll keep in the freezer for up to three months.

Cholate Mouse Tropical Bites

Serves: 12

Time: 45 Minutes

Calories: 174.67

Protein: 1.98 Grams

Fiber: 0.11 Grams

Fat: 13.75 Grams

Net Carbs: 1.02 Grams

Ingredients:

- Get out your molds and place them in the freezer. Take out a microwave safe bowl, and combine your coconut oil and dark chocolate together. Microwave it in ten second intervals, mixing well until melted. Make sure you don't burn your chocolate.
- Take a different bowl and whip your cream until it forms medium stiff peaks.
- Add your coconut and lemon zest into your cream by folding it in. reserve two thirds of your melted chocolate for your molds. Fold the other third into your cream mixture until your make a chocolate mousse. Store the mouse in the fridge so that it cools.
- Take your molds rom the freezer, pouring your chocolate in liberally. Move the tray around so that you get the molds covered on each side. It should be about three millimeters thick. If the chocolate is too hot, you won't be able to get a thick layer on all of your sides. Freeze it or fifteen minutes, and repeat the process if your chocolate is too thin.
- Take your cool mouse and then put it in your molds. Leave enough room at the top for the final layer of your chocolate.
- Cover each mold with chocolate to create a bottom, and then let it harden for fifteen minutes in the freezer. Some people like to add an extra little bit of lemon zest at the bottom.
- Serve frozen!

Pumpkin Fudge

Serves: 25

Time: 2 Hours 20 Minutes

Calories: 109.28

Protein: 1.2 Grams

Fiber: 2.63 Grams

Fat: 10.63 Grams

Net Carbs: 2.19 Grams

Ingredients:

- 1 Tablespoons Coconut Oil
- ¼ Teaspoon Ground Nutmeg
- 1 Cup Pumpkin Puree
- 1 Teaspoon Ground Cinnamon
- 1 ¾ Cps Coconut Butter

Directions:

1. Take an eight by eight baking pan, lining it with foil.
2. Spoon your coconut butter into a saucepan, placing it over low heat. Melt your coconut butter, and then remove it from heat. Stir in your spices and pumpkin, making sure it's mixed well. It's okay to have a grainy and thick texture right now.
3. Add in your coconut oil, and then mix well.
4. Spoon the mixture into your pan, and then put a piece of wax paper over the fudge, pressing it down.
5. Remove the wax paper, and then discard it. Place your fudge into the refrigerator for one to two hours. It should cool down and become firm.
6. Lift your fudge from the pan, and cut it into twenty-five squares. It'll store in the fridge or up to a week.

Conclusion

Now you have everything you need to get started with your five ingredient or less ketogenic cooking. There's no reason that getting healthy should be hard or time consuming, and with these recipes it's not! You'll be on your way to a happier, healthier you in no time at all. The ketogenic diet doesn't need to be difficult, and you won't have to break the bank to get tasty recipes that you can make on a busy schedule.

One more thing, if you've enjoyed this book, please post a review at the online retailer's website where you purchased the title from. It would be greatly appreciated.

Sign Up for Free Weekly Recipes, Tips and Tricks and more at:

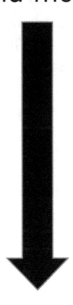

www.KetoDiet.coach

CPSIA information can be obtained
at www.ICGtesting.com
Printed in the USA
LVHW062141150919
631156LV00004B/492/P